Type 2 Diabetes Cookbook

Beginner's Quick & Easy Recipes for Delicious Diabetes Diets

300 Healthy

<u>Desserts</u>

for

Diabetic Wellness in 30 Minutes or Less

By

Lily Anders

Copyright Page

Ace East Publishing LLC
1401 21st Street
Suite R
Sacramento, CA 95811

ISBN: **978-1-963939-81-1**

First Edition

ACE EAST
PUBLISHING

Disclaimer Page

This cookbook is crafted to offer insightful information and recipes for those interested in managing Type 2 Diabetes through dietary choices. It is important to recognize that the authors and the publisher are not healthcare professionals. The suggestions and recipes contained within this book are not meant to replace professional medical advice, diagnoses, or treatments. Should you have any healthcare-related questions or concerns, particularly relating to Type 2 Diabetes management, we strongly advise consulting with your doctor or a qualified healthcare provider.

The culinary experiences and recommendations shared in this book stem from extensive research and the personal journey of exploring dietary approaches to Type 2 Diabetes management. These narratives and suggestions are intended for educational and motivational purposes only, aiming to enhance understanding and inspire positive lifestyle changes, not to serve as direct medical or nutritional prescriptions.

The author(s) and publisher expressly disclaim any liability for any adverse effects arising directly or indirectly from the use and application of the information contained in this cookbook. Moreover, given the specificity and medical relevance of the content, certain topics and dietary advice may not be suitable for all readers. It is advisable for caregivers and adults to review the content before sharing it with minors or individuals with particular sensitivities or health concerns.

In cases of medical emergencies or for immediate assistance with health issues, please reach out to a trusted healthcare professional or dial the emergency services number available in your locality.

The Entire Type 2 Diabetes Cookbook Series

Dive into a culinary revolution with the ***"Type 2 Diabetes Cookbook Series: Beginner's Quick & Easy Recipes for Delicious Diabetes Diets – 300 Health-Boosting Savory Meals for Diabetic Wellness in 30 Minutes or Less."***

Spread across six essential volumes – Breakfast, Lunch, Dinner, Desserts, Snacks, and Sauces, Dips, & Dressings – this series is your passport to a world where managing Type 2 Diabetes meets delicious innovation.

Each book is a treasure trove of hundreds of recipes, marrying the precision of nutritional science with the flair of culinary art. Designed for those on a diabetic diet, these recipes promise to transform your meals from bland to blissful without sacrificing flavor or health. Every dish, from energizing breakfasts to indulgent desserts, comes alive through vivid, full-color photographs, accompanied by foolproof instructions, cooking times, detailed ingredient lists, serving suggestions, and handy conversion charts.

But the journey doesn't end with tantalizing meals. These cookbooks are gateways to mastering diabetes management, offering insights into blood sugar balance, insulin functionality, and the art of carb counting. They stand as pillars of empowerment and knowledge, guiding you through the culinary and health aspects of diabetes with ease and enjoyment.

Embrace these cookbooks as more than mere collections of recipes; see them as companions in your journey toward diabetic wellness, bringing confidence, pleasure, and a burst of flavors into your daily life. Step into a world where managing diabetes is synonymous with culinary discovery and dietary joy. Welcome to your new kitchen adventure!

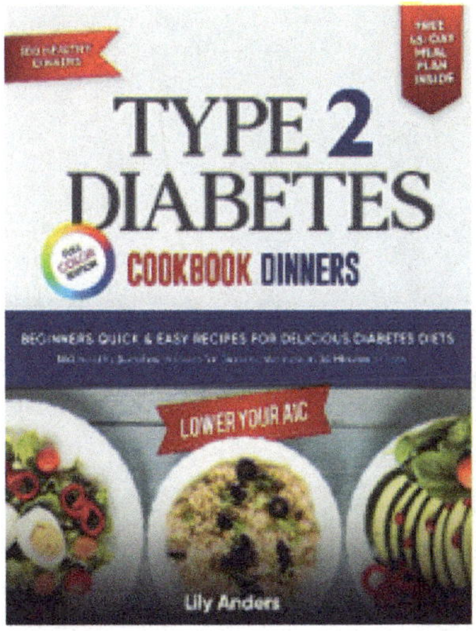
TYPE 2 DIABETES
COOKBOOK DINNERS
BEGINNERS QUICK & EASY RECIPES FOR DELICIOUS DIABETES DIETS
LOWER YOUR A1C
Lily Anders

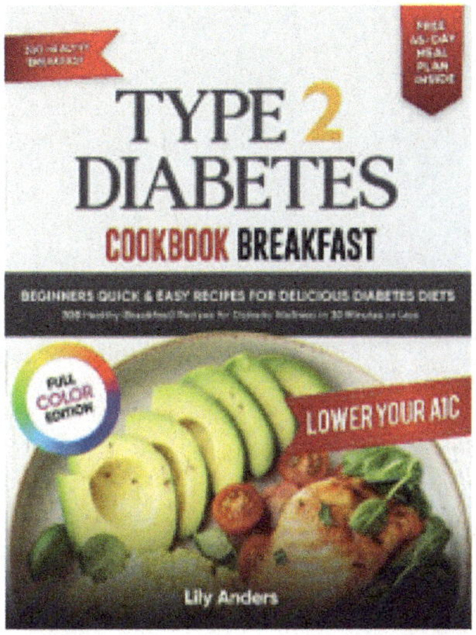
TYPE 2 DIABETES
COOKBOOK BREAKFAST
BEGINNERS QUICK & EASY RECIPES FOR DELICIOUS DIABETES DIETS
FULL COLOR EDITION
LOWER YOUR A1C
Lily Anders

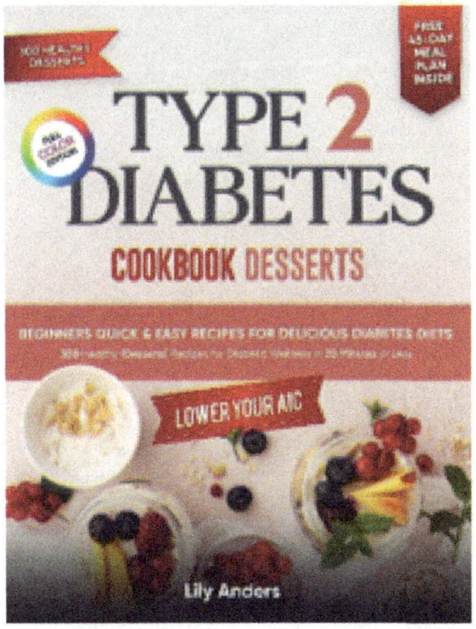
TYPE 2 DIABETES
COOKBOOK DESSERTS
LOWER YOUR A1C
Lily Anders

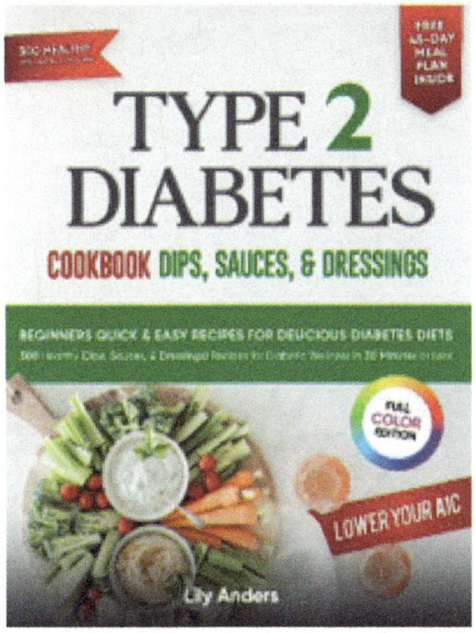
TYPE 2 DIABETES
COOKBOOK DIPS, SAUCES, & DRESSINGS
BEGINNERS QUICK & EASY RECIPES FOR DELICIOUS DIABETES DIETS
FULL COLOR EDITION
LOWER YOUR A1C
Lily Anders

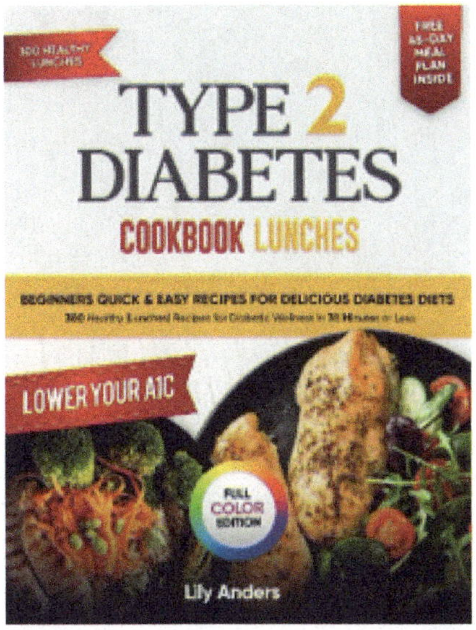
TYPE 2 DIABETES
COOKBOOK LUNCHES
BEGINNERS QUICK & EASY RECIPES FOR DELICIOUS DIABETES DIETS
LOWER YOUR A1C
FULL COLOR EDITION
Lily Anders

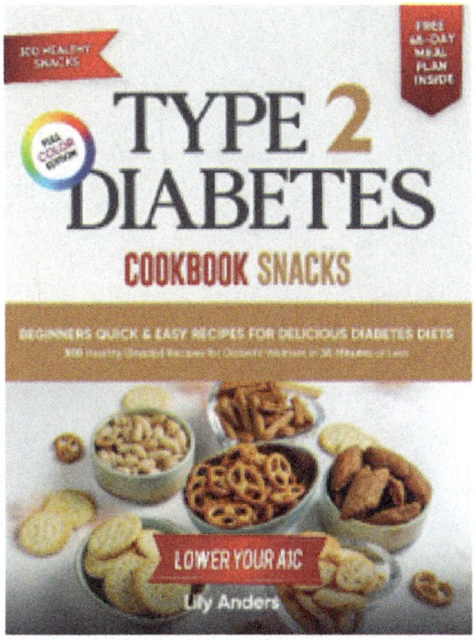
TYPE 2 DIABETES
COOKBOOK SNACKS
BEGINNERS QUICK & EASY RECIPES FOR DELICIOUS DIABETES DIETS
LOWER YOUR A1C
Lily Anders

Here's My Promise to You!

To jumpstart your journey toward healthier eating, here are the remaining

Listing of 200 Delicious & Diabetes-Friendly Dessert Recipes!

That's right—you now have access to a treasure trove of 200 additional diabetic recipes designed to help you enjoy flavorful, balanced meals while managing your blood sugar with confidence. These Dessert recipes will inspire you to create satisfying, nutritious meals with ease.

☞ CLICK THE LINK OR SCAN THE QR CODE TO DOWNLOAD YOUR FREE RECIPE COLLECTION!

Enjoy, and Happy Cooking!

The journey to better health starts with the right food choices, and this cookbook and it is here to support you every step of the way.

Thank you for trusting this guide, and here's to a flavorful, balanced, and empowered approach to managing Type 2 Diabetes!

You've got this! ☐☐✨

<<Click here to access your 45-day meal plan>>https://acrobat.adobe.com/id/urn:aaid:sc:VA6C2:448a7fa7-ffcd-4919-9d29-1c8e6bee62e9

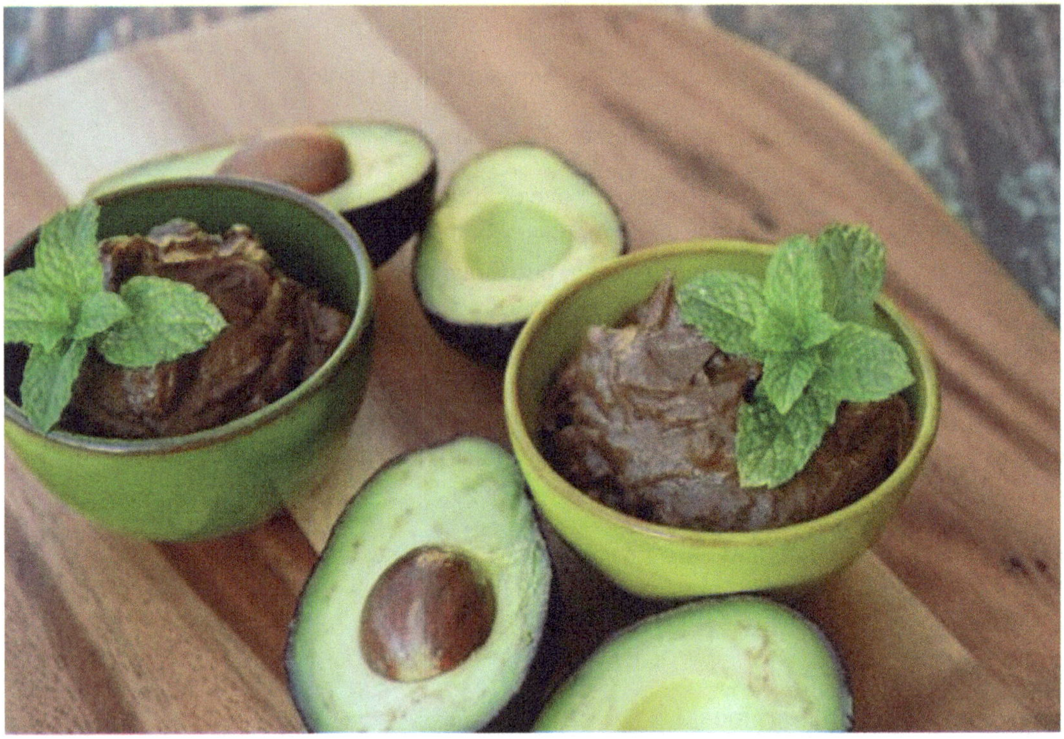

1. Sugar-Free Chocolate Avocado Mousse

Prep.Time: 10 min	**Cook Time:** 60 min	**Serving:** 4	**Beverage pairing:** Black Coffee

Ingredients:

- 2 ripe avocados
- 1/4 cup unsweetened cocoa powder
- 1/4 cup almond milk (unsweetened)
- 1/4 cup sugar-free sweetener (such as erythritol or stevia)
- 1 teaspoon vanilla extract
- A pinch of salt

Preparation:

1. Cut the avocados in half, remove the pit, and scoop out the flesh into a blender or food processor.
2. Add cocoa powder, almond milk, sugar-free sweetener, vanilla extract, and a pinch of salt to the blender.
3. Blend the ingredients until the mixture is smooth and creamy.
4. Taste and adjust sweetness as needed, adding more sweetener if desired.
5. Refrigerate the mousse for at least 1 hour before serving.

Nutrition Facts (per serving):

- Calories: 150
- Carbohydrates: 10g
- Fat: 12g
- Protein: 2g

Table of Contents

INTRODUCTION

Enjoying Sweetness with Confidence

For many people managing Type 2 Diabetes, dessert becomes the most emotionally charged part of eating. A diagnosis often turns sweetness into something forbidden, creating feelings of loss, frustration, or guilt. Celebrations feel different, cravings feel risky, and enjoyment can quietly disappear.

This book was written to change that experience.

Dessert does not need to be removed from your life in order to manage Type 2 Diabetes. What matters is how sweetness is approached, portioned, and balanced within your overall routine.

The Type 2 Diabetes Cookbook: Desserts focuses on thoughtful, diabetes-conscious desserts designed to satisfy without excess. These recipes are meant to restore enjoyment while supporting blood sugar balance and long-term consistency.

Desserts serve a different purpose than meals or snacks. They are often tied to emotion, tradition, and connection. Ignoring that role can make diabetes management feel restrictive and unsustainable. A more balanced approach allows room for enjoyment without creating unnecessary risk.

The good news is that diabetes-friendly desserts can still feel indulgent.

Inside this book, you will find dessert recipes that emphasize balance rather than deprivation. Each option is designed with portion awareness, ingredient quality, and pairing in mind. The goal is not to replicate high-sugar desserts exactly, but to create satisfying alternatives that feel intentional and enjoyable.

This cookbook is not about eating dessert every day or giving in to every craving. It is about knowing when and how dessert can fit into your life without fear.

You will not be asked to choose between enjoyment and responsibility. You will learn how to hold both at the same time.

Managing Type 2 Diabetes does not mean saying goodbye to sweetness. It means redefining it.

Welcome to a more confident, balanced way to enjoy dessert.

Chapter 1

Understanding Type 2 Diabetes and Sweet Foods

Sweet foods often feel like the first thing taken away after a Type 2 Diabetes diagnosis. Desserts are commonly associated with sugar, indulgence, and loss of control, which can create fear or avoidance. Understanding how sweet foods actually interact with the body helps replace fear with clarity.

Type 2 Diabetes affects how the body uses insulin, the hormone responsible for moving glucose from the bloodstream into the cells. When insulin does not function efficiently, glucose can remain in the blood longer than intended. Sweet foods, which often contain carbohydrates that are digested quickly, can influence this process more noticeably than other foods.

This does not mean dessert is automatically harmful. It means dessert requires intention.

Why Sweet Foods Feel Different

Sweet foods tend to digest faster than meals that contain protein, fiber, and fat. When eaten alone or in large portions, they can cause blood sugar levels to rise quickly. This rapid rise is often followed by a sharp drop, which may trigger fatigue, cravings, or discomfort.

For individuals managing Type 2 Diabetes, these fluctuations can feel more pronounced. This is why desserts are often viewed as risky or off-limits.

However, the issue is not sweetness itself. It is the combination of ingredients, portion size, and timing.

The Role of Dessert in a Balanced Routine

Desserts serve an emotional and social role that is different from meals or snacks. They are often enjoyed during celebrations, family gatherings, or moments of comfort. Ignoring this role can make diabetes management feel restrictive and isolating.

A balanced approach allows desserts to exist within a structured routine. When desserts are planned, portion-aware, and paired thoughtfully, they can be enjoyed without undermining blood sugar balance.

This approach supports both physical and emotional well-being.

Understanding Sugar Versus Carbohydrates

Sugar is one form of carbohydrate, but not all carbohydrates behave the same way. Desserts that rely heavily on refined sugars digest quickly and provide little nutritional support. Desserts that include fiber, protein, or healthy fats digest more slowly and create a gentler blood sugar response.

This distinction is important. It allows desserts to be reimagined rather than eliminated.

By focusing on ingredient quality and balance, desserts can become part of a supportive eating pattern rather than a source of disruption.

Removing Guilt from Dessert Choices

Guilt often leads to extremes, either complete avoidance or overeating. Neither supports long-term success.

This book encourages a neutral, informed approach to dessert. Understanding how sweet foods affect your body allows you to make choices without judgment.

When dessert is approached with intention, enjoyment becomes possible without regret.

Building Confidence Through Knowledge

As you learn how different dessert combinations affect your energy and blood sugar, confidence grows. You begin to recognize which options feel satisfying and which ones leave you uncomfortable.

This awareness allows you to enjoy dessert as a mindful choice rather than a reactive one.

In the next chapter, we will explore how blood sugar responds after desserts and why timing, pairing, and portion awareness make a meaningful difference.

Chapter 2

Blood Sugar Response to Desserts

Desserts affect blood sugar differently than meals or snacks, largely because they are often higher in carbohydrates and lower in protein or fiber. Understanding this response helps remove uncertainty and allows desserts to be enjoyed with greater confidence.

When dessert is eaten, carbohydrates are digested, and glucose enters the bloodstream. Insulin is released to help move this glucose into the cells. If this process happens too quickly, blood sugar levels can rise sharply and then fall just as rapidly. This pattern is often associated with fatigue, cravings, or discomfort.

For individuals managing Type 2 Diabetes, these fluctuations can feel more intense, especially when desserts are eaten without balance or intention.

Why Desserts Can Cause Rapid Changes

Many traditional desserts rely on refined sugars and flours, which digest quickly. Without protein, fiber, or fat to slow digestion, glucose enters the bloodstream rapidly.

This rapid entry can overwhelm the body's ability to manage blood sugar effectively, particularly in the evening or after large meals. The result is often a noticeable spike followed by a drop that leaves you feeling unsatisfied or uneasy.

The speed of digestion matters just as much as the amount of carbohydrates consumed.

The Importance of Pairing Desserts

Pairing desserts with other nutrients helps moderate blood sugar response. Protein, fiber, and healthy fats slow digestion and reduce the speed at which glucose enters the bloodstream.

Enjoying dessert after a balanced meal, rather than on an empty stomach, can also help stabilize blood sugar levels. When dessert is part of a structured eating pattern, the body is better prepared to handle it.

This approach allows desserts to feel more predictable and less disruptive.

Timing and Blood Sugar Stability

Timing plays a meaningful role in how desserts affect blood sugar. Desserts eaten earlier in the day, when activity levels are higher, may be processed differently than those eaten late at night.

Late evening desserts, especially those eaten alone, can lead to prolonged blood sugar elevations and interfere with sleep. Being mindful of timing helps desserts fit more comfortably into your routine.

This does not mean dessert must be avoided in the evening. It means portions and composition matter more during this time.

Recognizing Your Body's Signals

Each person responds differently to desserts. Some may tolerate certain combinations well, while others may notice discomfort or energy changes.

Paying attention to how you feel after dessert provides valuable information. Steady energy, comfort, and satisfaction are signs that balance is working. Fatigue, restlessness, or strong cravings may signal the need for adjustment.

Observation builds understanding without requiring strict rules.

Building Confidence Through Intention

When desserts are approached with intention, they become less intimidating. Understanding how blood sugar responds allows you to enjoy sweetness without fear or regret.

The dessert recipes in this book are designed to demonstrate how balance, pairing, and portion awareness can support enjoyment without disruption.

In the next chapter, we will focus on carbohydrates in desserts, how to include them thoughtfully, and how ingredient choices make a meaningful difference.

Chapter 3

Carbohydrates in Desserts Without Excess

Carbohydrates are an essential part of desserts, yet they are often the source of the greatest concern for individuals managing Type 2 Diabetes. Sugar, flour, and sweeteners can raise questions about safety and control, especially when desserts are associated with indulgence.

The goal with desserts is not to remove carbohydrates entirely. It is to understand how to include them in a way that supports balance and enjoyment without overwhelming the body.

Understanding Carbohydrate Sources in Desserts

Desserts commonly contain refined carbohydrates that digest quickly. White flour, added sugars, and syrups provide sweetness and texture but offer little resistance to digestion.

In contrast, desserts that incorporate fiber-rich ingredients such as nuts, seeds, whole grains, or fruit digest more slowly. These ingredients help moderate blood sugar response and add nutritional value.

Recognizing the difference between refined and fiber-containing carbohydrates allows desserts to be structured more thoughtfully.

Choosing Quality Over Quantity

The quality of carbohydrates in desserts often matters more than the quantity alone. Smaller portions of well-chosen ingredients can provide satisfaction without excess.

Using ingredients that offer natural sweetness or added texture allows desserts to feel indulgent while remaining balanced. This approach reduces the need for large amounts of refined sugars.

When desserts emphasize quality, portions naturally become more manageable.

The Role of Portion Awareness in Desserts

Portion size is especially important with desserts. Even balanced ingredients can create blood sugar challenges when portions are large.

Desserts are meant to be enjoyed in moderation. Smaller servings can still feel satisfying when flavors are rich, and textures are thoughtful.

Portion awareness helps desserts remain a positive experience rather than a source of discomfort or regret.

Pairing Desserts for Balance

Pairing desserts with protein or healthy fats helps slow digestion and reduce blood sugar spikes. Ingredients such as nuts, seeds, yogurt, or cheese can complement sweet flavors while supporting balance.

Desserts enjoyed as part of a meal, rather than alone, often feel more stable and predictable. This pairing approach allows sweetness to fit naturally into a balanced routine.

Redefining Dessert Expectations

Desserts do not need to mimic traditional high-sugar treats exactly to be enjoyable. Redefining expectations allows room for creativity and balance.

When desserts are viewed as intentional choices rather than forbidden indulgences, they become easier to manage.

The recipes in this book demonstrate how carbohydrates can be included thoughtfully, allowing desserts to remain enjoyable without excess.

In the next chapter, we will focus on smart dessert shopping, helping you choose ingredients that support balanced, diabetes-conscious desserts.

Chapter 4

Smart Dessert Shopping

Dessert shopping often feels more complicated than it needs to be. Labels can be confusing, ingredients unfamiliar, and marketing messages misleading. For individuals managing Type 2 Diabetes, these challenges can make dessert feel risky or overwhelming before it even reaches the kitchen.

Smart dessert shopping removes much of that uncertainty and restores confidence.

Shopping With Intention, Not Restriction

Dessert shopping is not about avoiding entire sections of the store. It is about choosing ingredients that support balance, portion awareness, and satisfaction.

Focusing on whole, recognizable ingredients helps simplify decisions. Nuts, seeds, unsweetened cocoa, plain yogurt, fruits, and whole grains form a strong foundation for diabetes-conscious desserts.

When ingredients are chosen intentionally, desserts become easier to plan and enjoy.

Navigating Sweeteners and Baking Ingredients

Sweeteners are a common source of confusion. Many desserts rely on refined sugars that digest quickly and contribute to blood sugar spikes.

When shopping, look for alternatives that allow sweetness to be controlled more carefully. Using smaller amounts of sweeteners or choosing ingredients that provide natural sweetness helps reduce excess.

Flours and baking mixes also deserve attention. Products made with refined white flour often digest rapidly. Whole grain or alternative flours that contain fiber provide a more balanced option when used thoughtfully.

Reading Labels Without Overwhelm

Label reading does not need to be complicated. Start by looking at ingredient lists rather than marketing claims.

Shorter ingredient lists with recognizable components are often better choices. Be mindful of added sugars, syrups, or highly processed ingredients that appear early in the list.

Nutrition labels can provide additional insight, but they are most helpful when used as a guide rather than a strict rulebook.

Choosing Desserts for Flexibility

Dessert ingredients should support flexibility and creativity. Items that can be used in multiple recipes reduce waste and simplify planning.

Frozen fruits, nuts, seeds, and baking staples with longer shelf lives make it easier to prepare desserts without frequent shopping trips.

Keeping a small selection of reliable dessert ingredients on hand allows you to enjoy sweetness without impulse purchases.

Making Dessert Shopping Sustainable

Effective dessert shopping supports long-term habits. When ingredients are familiar and dependable, dessert preparation feels approachable rather than intimidating.

Over time, dessert shopping becomes quicker and more intuitive, and desserts feel like a natural, balanced part of your routine.

In the next chapter, we will explore preparation strategies that make desserts easier to prepare, helping you enjoy them without unnecessary effort or stress.

Chapter 5

Prep Strategies for Balanced Desserts

Desserts feel far more manageable when preparation is simple and intentional. When recipes are overly complex or time-consuming, desserts can become an occasional indulgence driven by impulse rather than a thoughtful choice. For individuals managing Type 2 Diabetes, preparation strategies help desserts remain balanced, portion-aware, and stress-free.

Preparation does not need to be elaborate. Small, practical steps can make a meaningful difference.

Preparing Dessert Components Ahead of Time

Preparing certain elements in advance reduces effort and encourages consistency. Chopping nuts, portioning baking ingredients, or preparing simple bases allows desserts to come together quickly when needed.

Items such as fruit compotes, yogurt bases, or pre-measured dry ingredients can be stored and used across multiple recipes. These components support balance while reducing preparation time.

Advance preparation also helps avoid last-minute choices that may be less supportive.

Choosing Simple, Repeatable Techniques

Dessert preparation benefits from simplicity. No-bake recipes, small-batch baking, and one-bowl methods reduce complexity and cleanup.

These techniques make desserts more accessible and less intimidating. When preparation feels manageable, desserts are more likely to be enjoyed intentionally rather than avoided or overindulged.

Simple methods also make portion control easier.

Planning Desserts With Purpose

Desserts are best enjoyed when planned rather than reactive. Deciding in advance when dessert will be included helps remove guilt and reduce impulsive eating.

Planning desserts around meals or occasions allows you to enjoy them with greater awareness. This approach supports both satisfaction and balance.

Preparation supports planning by ensuring ingredients and portions are ready when desired.

Storing Desserts for Portion Awareness

How desserts are stored can influence portion size. Storing desserts in individual servings or small containers makes it easier to enjoy an appropriate amount without overconsumption.

Freezing portions or refrigerating desserts in clearly labeled containers helps maintain structure and flexibility. This allows desserts to be enjoyed over time rather than all at once.

Creating a Sustainable Dessert Routine

Desserts become easier to manage when they are part of a routine rather than an exception. A balanced dessert routine respects both enjoyment and responsibility.

When preparation is simple and portions are planned, desserts can be included without stress.

In the next chapter, we will focus on portion awareness for desserts, helping you enjoy sweetness without excess and maintain confidence in your choices.

Chapter 6

Portion Awareness for Enjoyable Desserts

Portion size is one of the most important factors in enjoying desserts while managing Type 2 Diabetes. Even thoughtfully prepared desserts can disrupt blood sugar balance when portions are larger than intended. Portion awareness helps desserts remain a positive, satisfying experience rather than a source of concern.

Portion awareness is not about deprivation. It is about choosing an amount that allows you to enjoy sweetness without discomfort, guilt, or unintended blood sugar changes.

Why Dessert Portions Matter

Desserts are typically higher in carbohydrates than other foods. Larger portions can cause blood sugar levels to rise more quickly and remain elevated longer, especially when desserts are eaten alone or late in the day.

Smaller portions allow the body to process carbohydrates more gradually, reducing the likelihood of spikes and crashes. When desserts are portioned intentionally, enjoyment often increases because the experience feels controlled and deliberate.

Recognizing Satisfying Portions

A satisfying dessert portion is often smaller than expected. Rich flavors, varied textures, and thoughtful ingredients help smaller servings feel complete.

Using small bowls, plates, or ramekins can support portion awareness visually. Serving desserts individually rather than from a shared container also helps maintain balance.

Taking time to eat slowly and without distraction improves satisfaction and helps you recognize when enough is enough.

Common Dessert Portion Challenges

Desserts are often associated with celebration or emotional comfort, which can lead to larger portions or repeated servings. Eating directly from baking dishes or large containers makes it easier to lose track of portion size.

Another common challenge is saving dessert until late evening, when hunger and fatigue are highest. Being mindful of timing and portion size can help prevent overeating.

Recognizing these patterns allows for gentle adjustments rather than rigid rules.

Adjusting Portions Without Losing Enjoyment

If desserts leave you feeling uncomfortable or unsatisfied, portion size or composition may need adjustment. Reducing portion size slightly or pairing dessert with protein or healthy fats can improve balance.

Flexibility is key. Some occasions may allow for slightly larger portions, while everyday enjoyment may call for smaller servings. This adaptability supports long-term consistency.

Building Confidence Through Consistency

Over time, portion awareness becomes intuitive. As you repeat balanced dessert experiences, your body responds more predictably, and confidence grows.

The dessert recipes in this book are designed with portion awareness in mind, helping remove guesswork while preserving enjoyment.

In the next section, we will transition into the dessert recipes, where these principles come together in thoughtful, satisfying ways.

Enjoying Dessert with Intention

The guidance you have explored in this section is meant to restore confidence, not create hesitation. Understanding how desserts interact with blood sugar, learning to include carbohydrates thoughtfully, and developing practical habits around shopping, preparation, and portion awareness all serve one purpose. . . to help you enjoy sweetness without fear.

Now it is time to put those principles into practice.

The dessert recipes that follow are designed to balance enjoyment with responsibility. Each recipe emphasizes thoughtful ingredients, manageable portions, and combinations that support blood sugar stability while still feeling indulgent. These desserts are meant to be savored, not rushed, and enjoyed with intention rather than guilt.

You do not need to prepare every recipe or save them only for special occasions. Choose desserts that fit your preferences, your schedule, and your goals. Some moments may call for something light and simple, while others may invite a more deliberate treat. Both are supported here.

As you explore the recipes, pay attention to how different desserts make you feel, both during and after enjoyment. Use that awareness to guide future choices and refine what works best for you.

This section is not about restriction or perfection. It is about creating space for sweetness within a balanced life.

Let these recipes remind you that managing Type 2 Diabetes can include pleasure, comfort, and confidence.

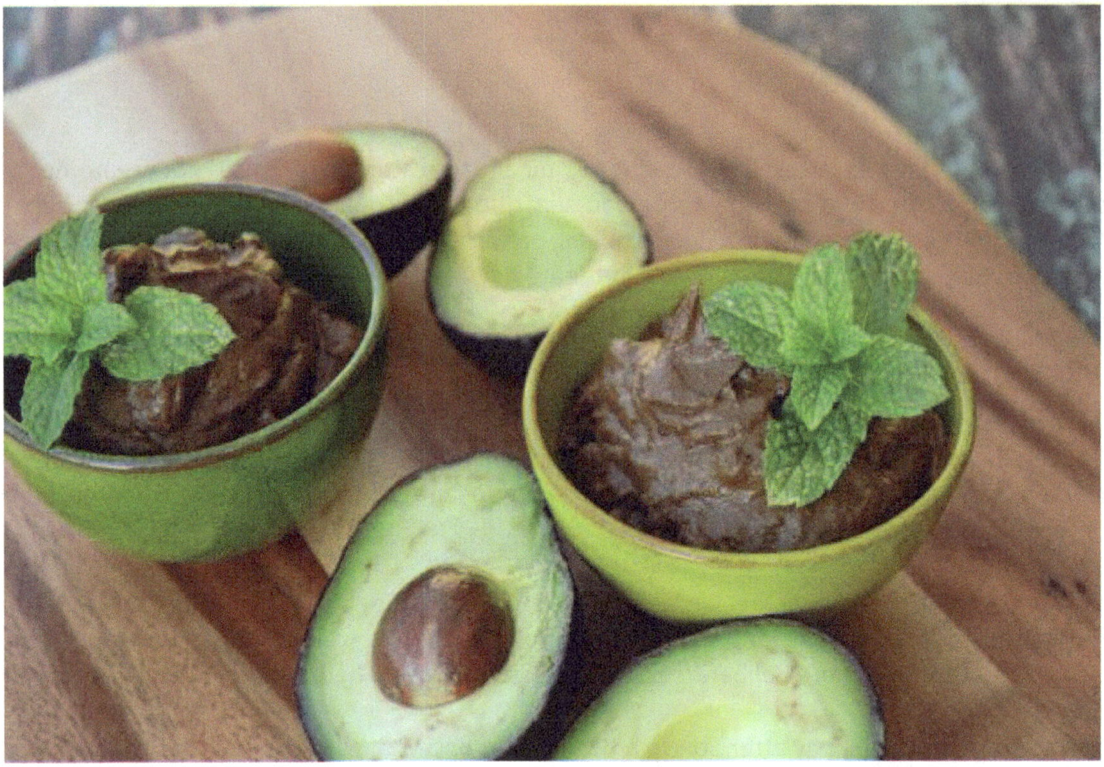

1. Sugar-Free Chocolate Avocado Mousse

Prep.Time: 10 min

Cook Time: 60 min

Serving: 4

Beverage pairing: Black Coffee

Ingredients:

- 2 ripe avocados
- 1/4 cup unsweetened cocoa powder
- 1/4 cup almond milk (unsweetened)
- 1/4 cup sugar-free sweetener (such as erythritol or stevia)
- 1 teaspoon vanilla extract
- A pinch of salt

Preparation:

1. Cut the avocados in half, remove the pit, and scoop out the flesh into a blender or food processor.
2. Add cocoa powder, almond milk, sugar-free sweetener, vanilla extract, and a pinch of salt to the blender.
3. Blend the ingredients until the mixture is smooth and creamy.
4. Taste and adjust sweetness as needed, adding more sweetener if desired.
5. Refrigerate the mousse for at least 1 hour before serving.

Nutrition Facts (per serving):

- Calories: 150
- Carbohydrates: 10g
- Fat: 12g
- Protein: 2g

2. Almond Flour Blueberry Muffins

Prep.Time:	Cook Time:	Serving:	Beverage pairing:
15 min	20 min	12	Peppermint tea

Ingredients:

- 2 cups almond flour
- 1/4 cup coconut flour
- 1 teaspoon baking powder
- 1/2 teaspoon baking soda
- 1/4 teaspoon salt
- 1/4 cup melted coconut oil
- 1/4 cup unsweetened almond milk
- 3 large eggs
- 1/4 cup sugar-free sweetener (erythritol or stevia)
- 1 teaspoon vanilla extract
- 1 cup fresh or frozen blueberries

Preparation:

1. Preheat the oven to 350°F (175°C) and line a muffin tin with paper liners.
2. In a large bowl, whisk together almond flour, coconut flour, baking powder, baking soda, and salt.
3. In a separate bowl, whisk together melted coconut oil, almond milk, eggs, sugar-free sweetener, and vanilla extract.
4. Add the wet ingredients to the dry ingredients and stir until well combined.
5. Gently fold in the blueberries.
6. Spoon the batter into the muffin cups, filling each about 2/3 full.
7. Bake for 20-25 minutes or until a toothpick inserted into the center comes out clean.
8. Allow the muffins to cool in the tin for 10 minutes before transferring them to a wire rack to cool completely.

Nutrition Facts (per serving):

- Calories: 180
- Carbohydrates: 8g
- Fat: 14g
- Protein: 6g

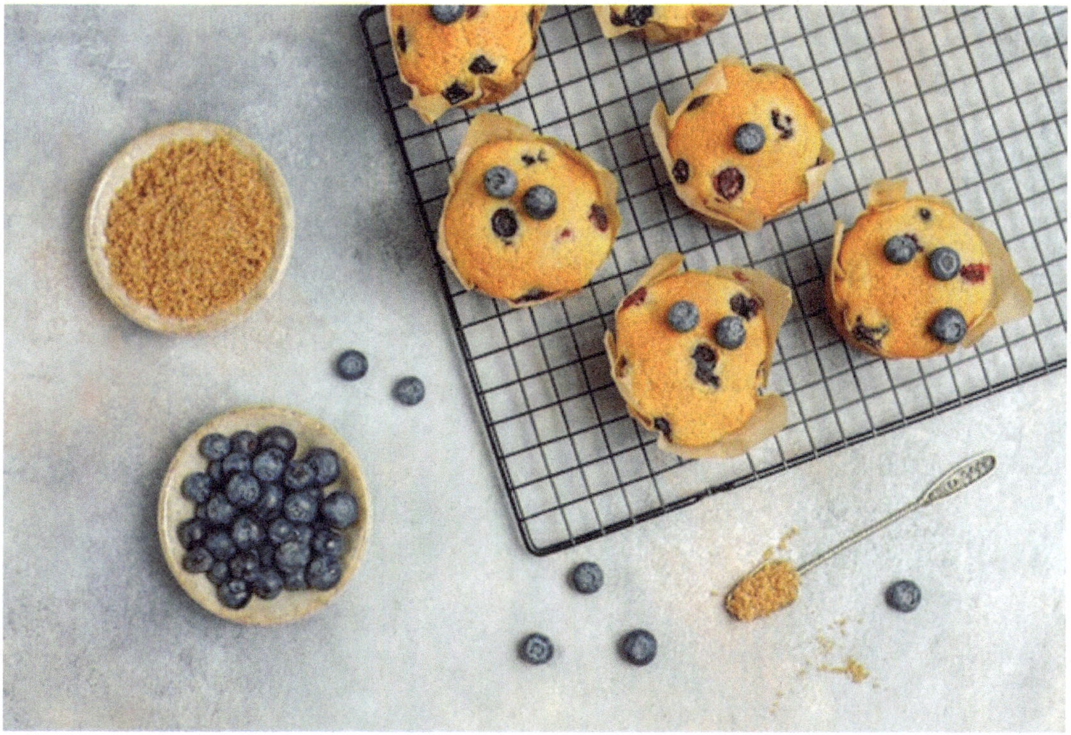

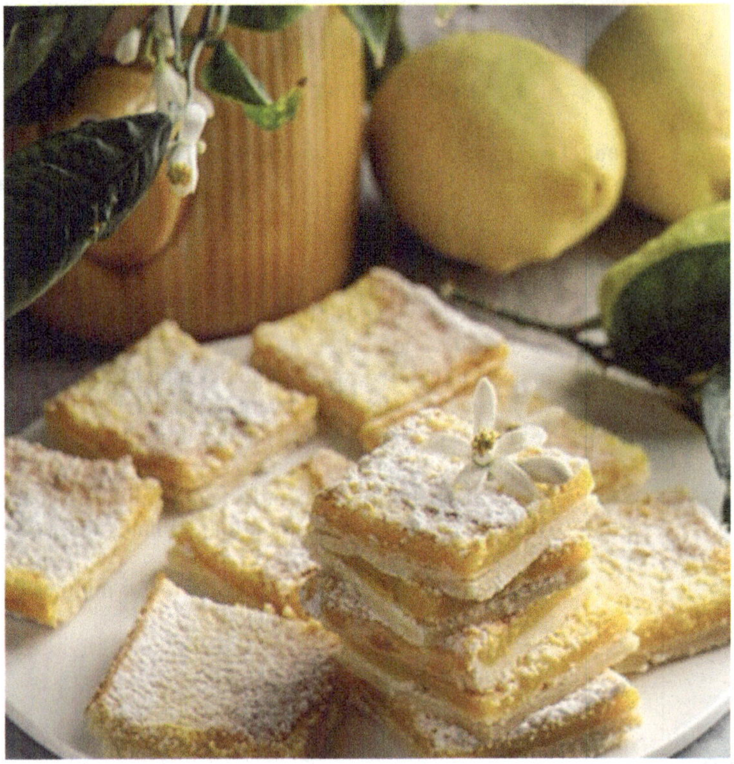

3. Stevia-Sweetened Lemon Bars

Prep.Time:	Cook Time:	Serving:	Beverage pairing:
15 min	40 min	12	Iced Tea

Ingredients:

- 1 cup almond flour
- 1/4 cup coconut flour
- 1/4 cup melted coconut oil
- 1/4 cup powdered stevia
- 4 large eggs
- 1 cup fresh lemon juice
- Zest of 2 lemons
- 1/2 cup powdered stevia
- 1/4 cup coconut flour
- 1/2 teaspoon baking powder
- A pinch of salt

Preparation:

1. Preheat the oven to 350°F (175°C) and line a baking dish with parchment paper.
2. In a bowl, combine almond flour, coconut flour, melted coconut oil, and powdered stevia. Press the mixture into the bottom of the prepared baking dish to form the crust.
3. Bake the crust for 10-12 minutes or until golden brown.
4. Meanwhile, prepare the lemon filling by whisking together eggs, lemon juice, lemon zest, powdered stevia, coconut flour, baking powder, and a pinch of salt.
5. Pour the lemon filling over the baked crust and return it to the oven for another 20-25 minutes, or until set.
6. Allow the lemon bars to cool completely before cutting into squares.

Nutrition Facts (per serving):

- Calories: 120
- Carbohydrates: 7g
- Fat: 9g
- Protein: 3g

4. Cinnamon Baked Apples

Prep.Time:	Cook Time:	Serving:	Beverage pairing:
10 min	25 min	4	Herbal tea

Ingredients:

- 4 medium-sized apples, cored and sliced
- 1 tablespoon melted coconut oil
- 1 teaspoon ground cinnamon
- 1/4 teaspoon nutmeg
- 1/4 cup chopped walnuts (optional)
- 1 tablespoon sugar-free sweetener (erythritol or stevia)

Preparation:

1. Preheat the oven to 375°F (190°C).
2. In a bowl, toss the apple slices with melted coconut oil, ground cinnamon, nutmeg, chopped walnuts (if using), and sugar-free sweetener.
3. Transfer the coated apples to a baking dish.
4. Bake for 20-25 minutes or until the apples are tender.
5. Serve warm, optionally topped with a dollop of sugar-free whipped cream.

Nutrition Facts (per serving):

- Calories: 120
- Carbohydrates: 18g
- Fat: 6g
- Protein: 1g

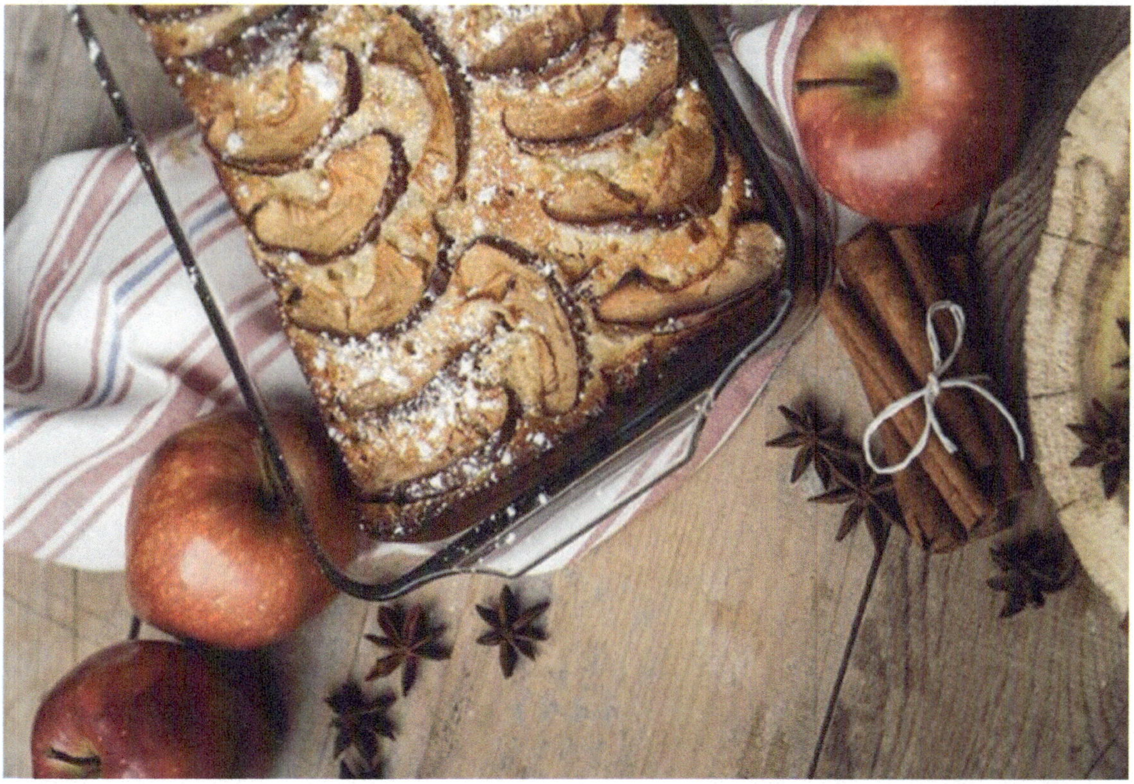

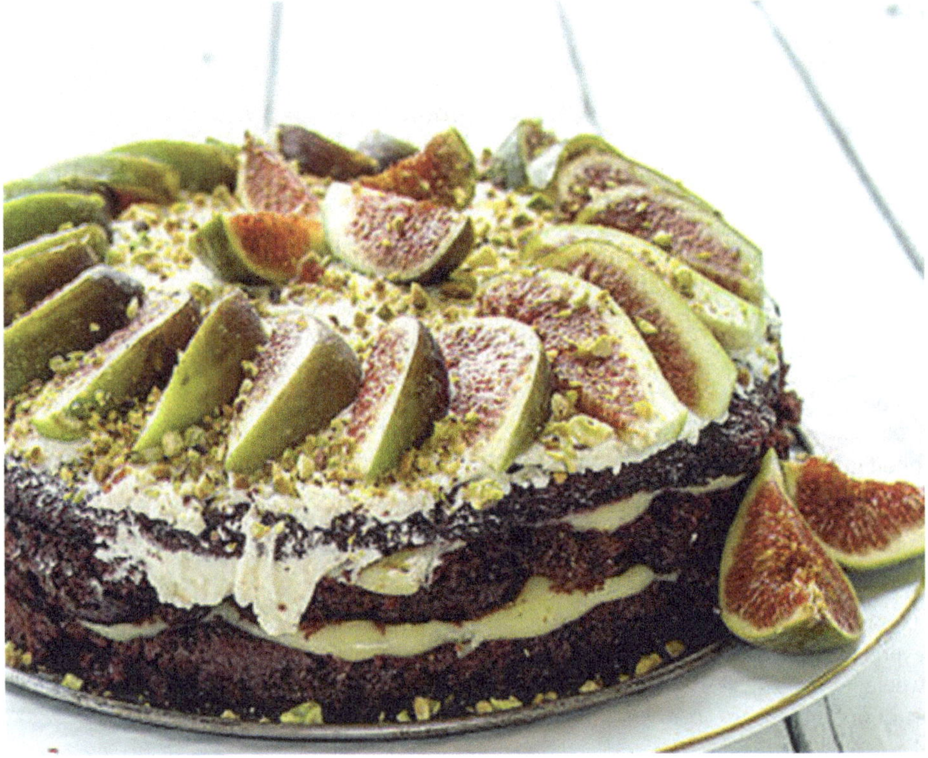

5. Almond Flour Fig and Pistachio Cake

Prep.Time: 15 min

Cook Time: 35 min

Serving: 8

Beverage pairing: Tea

Ingredients:

- 1 1/2 cups almond flour
- 1/2 cup coconut flour
- 1 tsp baking powder
- 1/2 tsp baking soda
- 1/4 tsp salt
- 1/2 cup unsweetened applesauce
- 1/4 cup melted coconut oil
- 1/4 cup honey or maple syrup
- 3 large eggs
- 1 tsp vanilla extract
- 1/2 cup chopped dried figs
- 1/4 cup chopped pistachios

Preparation:

1. Preheat oven to 350°F (175°C). Grease and line a 9-inch round cake pan.
2. Whisk almond flour, coconut flour, baking powder, baking soda, and salt in a bowl.
3. In another bowl, mix applesauce, coconut oil, honey/maple syrup, eggs, and vanilla.
4. Combine wet and dry ingredients, then fold in figs and pistachios.
5. Pour batter into the pan and bake for 30-35 minutes.
6. Cool in the pan for 10 minutes, then transfer to a wire rack to cool completely.
7. Garnish with sliced figs and pistachios if desired.
8. Serve and enjoy!

Nutrition Facts (per serving):

- Calories: 250
- Carbohydrates: 20g
- Fat: 20g
- Protein: 8g

6. Dark Chocolate-Dipped Strawberries

Prep.Time:	Cook Time:	Serving:	Beverage pairing:
15 min	30 min	4	Almond Milk

Ingredients:

- 1 cup dark chocolate chips (sugar-free or at least 70% cocoa)
- 1 pound fresh strawberries, washed and dried

Preparation:

1. Line a tray or plate with parchment paper.
2. In a microwave-safe bowl, melt the dark chocolate chips in 30-second intervals, stirring between each interval until smooth.
3. Hold each strawberry by the green stem and dip it into the melted chocolate, swirling to coat evenly.
4. Place the dipped strawberries on the parchment paper.
5. Refrigerate for at least 30 minutes or until the chocolate is set.

Nutrient Facts (per serving - 4 strawberries):

- Calories: 120
- Carbohydrates: 15g
- Fat: 8g
- Protein: 2g

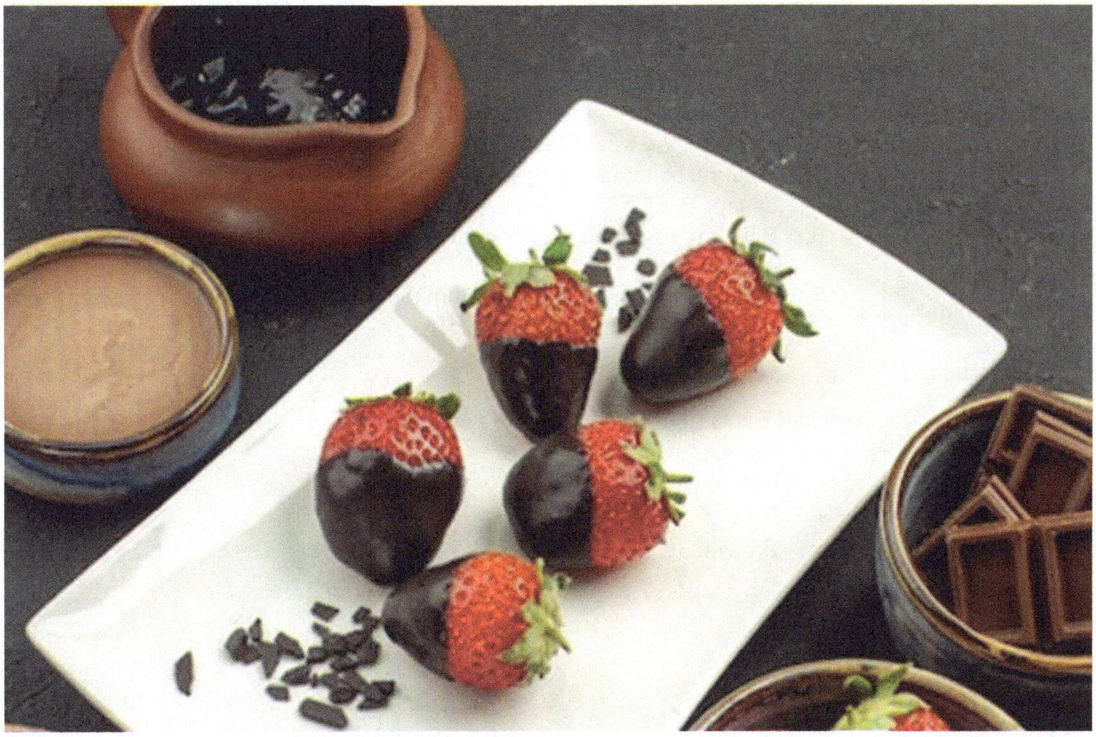

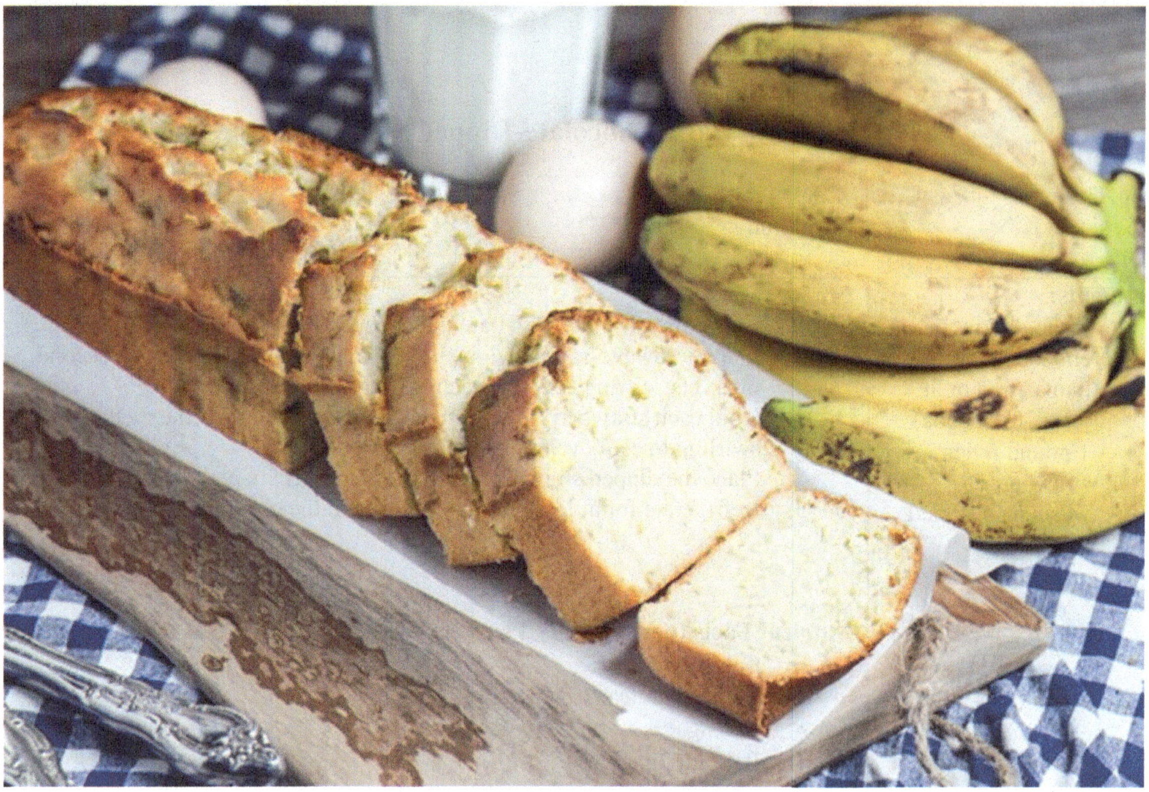

7. Coconut Flour Banana Bread

Prep.Time: 15 min

Cook Time: 40 min

Serving: 12

Beverage pairing: Black Coffee

Ingredients:

- 3 ripe bananas, mashed
- 3 large eggs
- 1/4 cup melted coconut oil
- 1/4 cup unsweetened almond milk
- 1 teaspoon vanilla extract
- 1/2 cup coconut flour
- 1 teaspoon baking powder
- 1/2 teaspoon baking soda
- 1/2 teaspoon ground cinnamon
- A pinch of salt
- Chopped nuts for topping (optional)

Preparation:

1. Preheat the oven to 350°F (175°C). Grease a loaf pan.
2. In a large bowl, mash the ripe bananas and add eggs, melted coconut oil, almond milk, and vanilla extract. Mix well.
3. In a separate bowl, whisk together coconut flour, baking powder, baking soda, ground cinnamon, and a pinch of salt.
4. Combine the wet and dry ingredients, stirring until just combined.
5. Pour the batter into the prepared loaf pan. Optionally, sprinkle chopped nuts on top.
6. Bake for 40-45 minutes or until a toothpick inserted into the center comes out clean.
7. Allow the banana bread to cool in the pan for 10 minutes before transferring it to a wire rack to cool completely.

Nutrient Facts (per slice - 12 slices per loaf):

- Calories: 120
- Carbohydrates: 10g
- Fat: 7g
- Protein: 3g

8. Sugar-Free Raspberry Sorbet

Prep.Time:	**Cook Time:**	**Serving:**	**Beverage pairing:**
10 min	0 min	6	Iced Tea

Ingredients:

- 3 cups frozen raspberries
- 1/4 cup water
- 1/4 cup sugar-free sweetener (erythritol or stevia)
- 1 tablespoon fresh lemon juice

Preparation:

1. In a blender or food processor, combine frozen raspberries, water, sugar-free sweetener, and fresh lemon juice.
2. Blend until smooth, scraping down the sides as needed.
3. Taste and adjust sweetness if necessary, adding more sweetener or lemon juice.
4. Transfer the sorbet mixture to a shallow dish and freeze for at least 2 hours.
5. Before serving, let the sorbet soften for a few minutes at room temperature and then scoop into bowls.

Nutrient Facts (per serving - 1/2 cup):

- Calories: 40
- Carbohydrates: 8g
- Fat: 0g
- Protein: 1g

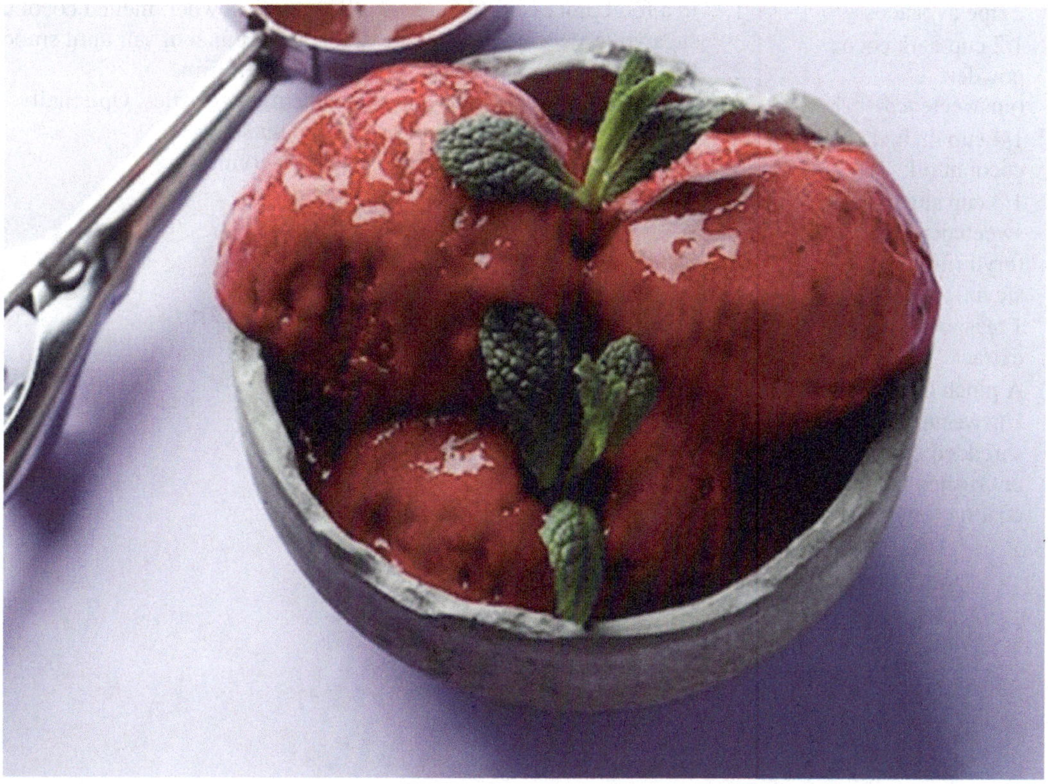

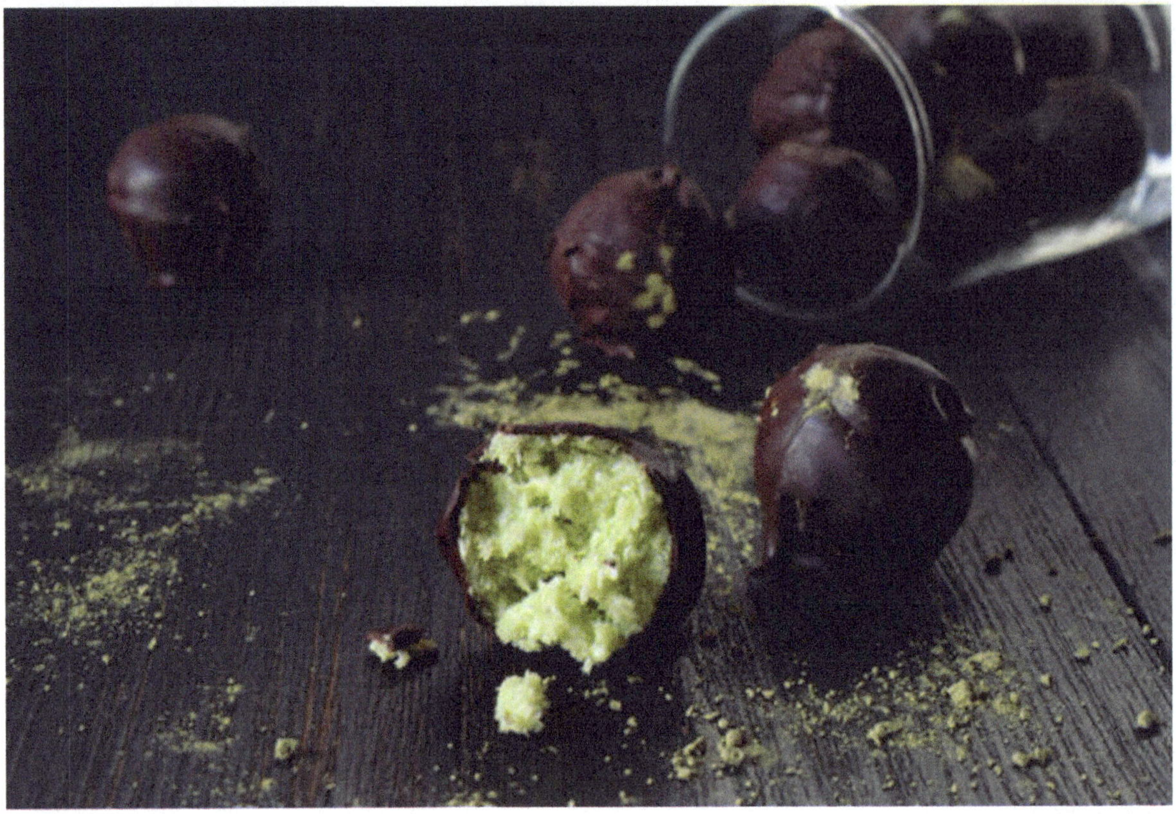

9. Avocado Chocolate Truffles

Prep.Time: 15 min

Cook Time: 0 min

Serving: 12

Beverage pairing: Herbal Tea

Ingredients:

- 2 ripe avocados
- 1/2 cup dark cocoa powder (unsweetened)
- 1/4 cup melted coconut oil
- 1/4 cup sugar-free sweetener (erythritol or stevia)
- 1 teaspoon vanilla extract
- A pinch of salt
- Unsweetened shredded coconut or crushed nuts for coating (optional)

Preparation:

1. In a food processor, blend avocados, cocoa powder, melted coconut oil, sugar-free sweetener, vanilla extract, and a pinch of salt until smooth.
2. Refrigerate the mixture for 1-2 hours or until firm.
3. Scoop out small portions and shape them into truffles. Optionally, roll the truffles in shredded coconut or crushed nuts.
4. Refrigerate again for 30 minutes before serving.

Nutrient Facts (per truffle - makes approximately 12):

- Calories: 80
- Carbohydrates: 6g
- Fat: 6g
- Protein: 2g

10. Greek Yogurt Parfait with Berries

Prep.Time: 5 min

Cook Time: 0 min

Serving: 1

Beverage pairing: Green Tea

Ingredients:

- 1 cup Greek yogurt (unsweetened)
- 1/2 cup mixed berries (strawberries, blueberries, raspberries)
- 1 tablespoon sugar-free granola
- 1 tablespoon chopped nuts (almonds or walnuts)
- 1 teaspoon honey or sugar-free sweetener (optional)

Preparation:

1. In a glass or bowl, layer Greek yogurt, mixed berries, sugar-free granola, and chopped nuts.
2. Repeat the layers until the container is filled.
3. Optionally, drizzle honey or sugar-free sweetener on top.
4. Serve immediately.

Nutrient Facts (per serving):

- Calories: 150
- Carbohydrates: 15g
- Fat: 7g
- Protein: 12g

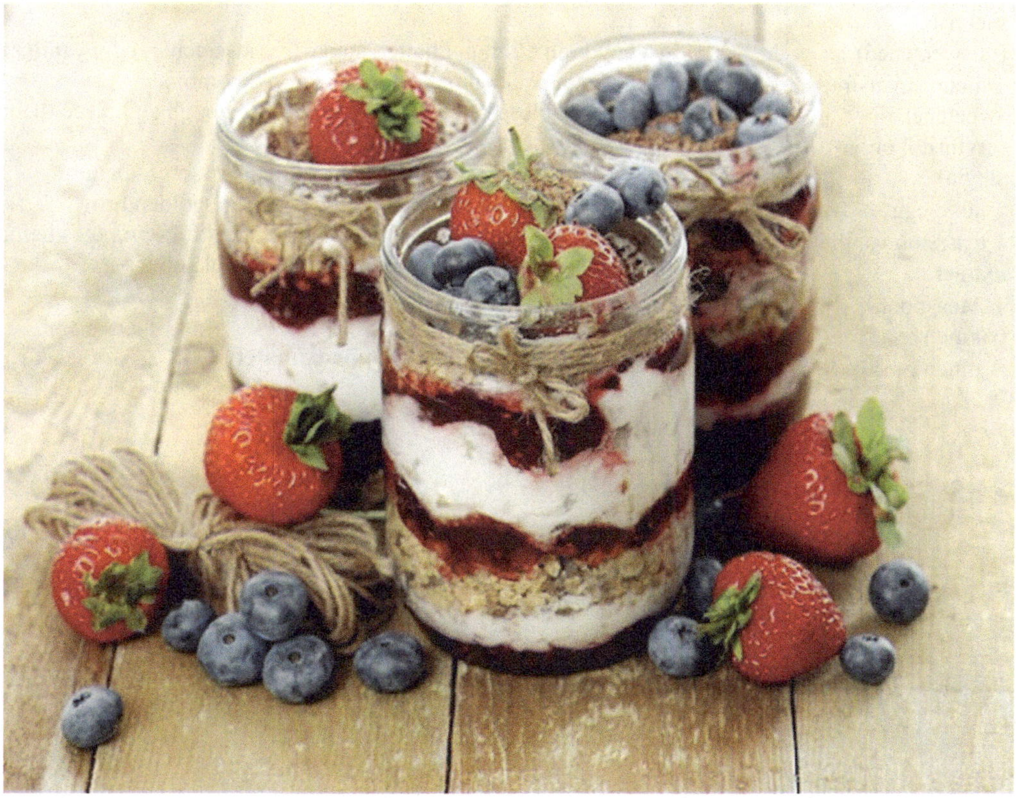

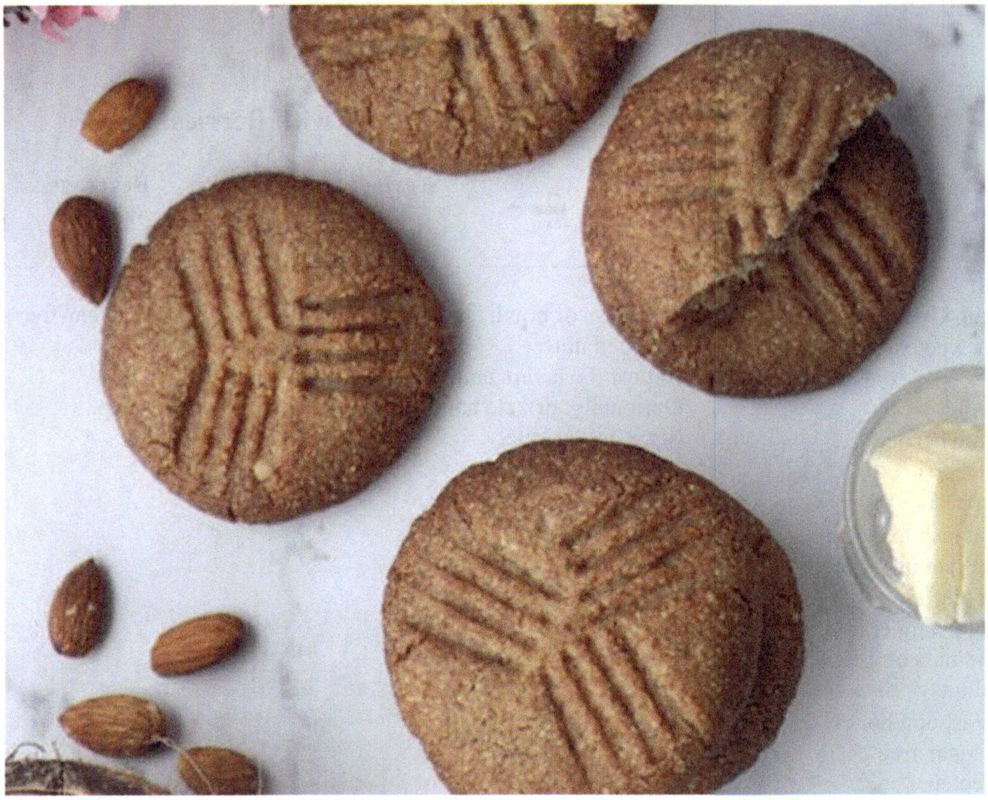

11. Almond Butter Cookies

Prep.Time: 10 min | **Cook Time:** 12 min | **Serving:** 12 | **Beverage pairing:** Herbal Tea

Ingredients:

- 1 cup almond butter (unsweetened)
- 1/4 cup sugar-free sweetener (erythritol or stevia)
- 1 large egg
- 1 teaspoon vanilla extract
- 1/2 teaspoon baking soda
- A pinch of salt

Preparation:

1. Preheat the oven to 350°F (175°C) and line a baking sheet with parchment paper.
2. In a bowl, mix almond butter, sugar-free sweetener, egg, vanilla extract, baking soda, and a pinch of salt until well combined.
3. Scoop out tablespoon-sized portions of the dough and place them on the prepared baking sheet.
4. Flatten each cookie with a fork, creating a crisscross pattern.
5. Bake for 10-12 minutes or until the edges are golden brown.
6. Allow the cookies to cool on the baking sheet for 5 minutes before transferring them to a wire rack to cool completely.

Nutrient Facts (per cookie - makes approximately 12):

- Calories: 120
- Carbohydrates: 4g
- Fat: 10g
- Protein: 4g

12. Cocoa-Dusted Almonds

Prep.Time:	Cook Time:	Serving:	Beverage pairing:
10 min	0 min	4	Black Coffee

Ingredients:

- 1 cup raw almonds
- 1 tablespoon cocoa powder (unsweetened)
- 1 tablespoon sugar-free sweetener (erythritol or stevia)
- A pinch of salt

Preparation:

1. In a dry skillet over medium heat, toast the almonds until fragrant, about 5-7 minutes. Stir frequently to prevent burning.
2. In a bowl, combine cocoa powder, sugar-free sweetener, and a pinch of salt.
3. Toss the toasted almonds in the cocoa mixture until well coated.
4. Allow the almonds to cool before serving.

Nutrient Facts (per serving - 1/4 cup):

- Calories: 150
- Carbohydrates: 5g
- Fat: 13g
- Protein: 5g

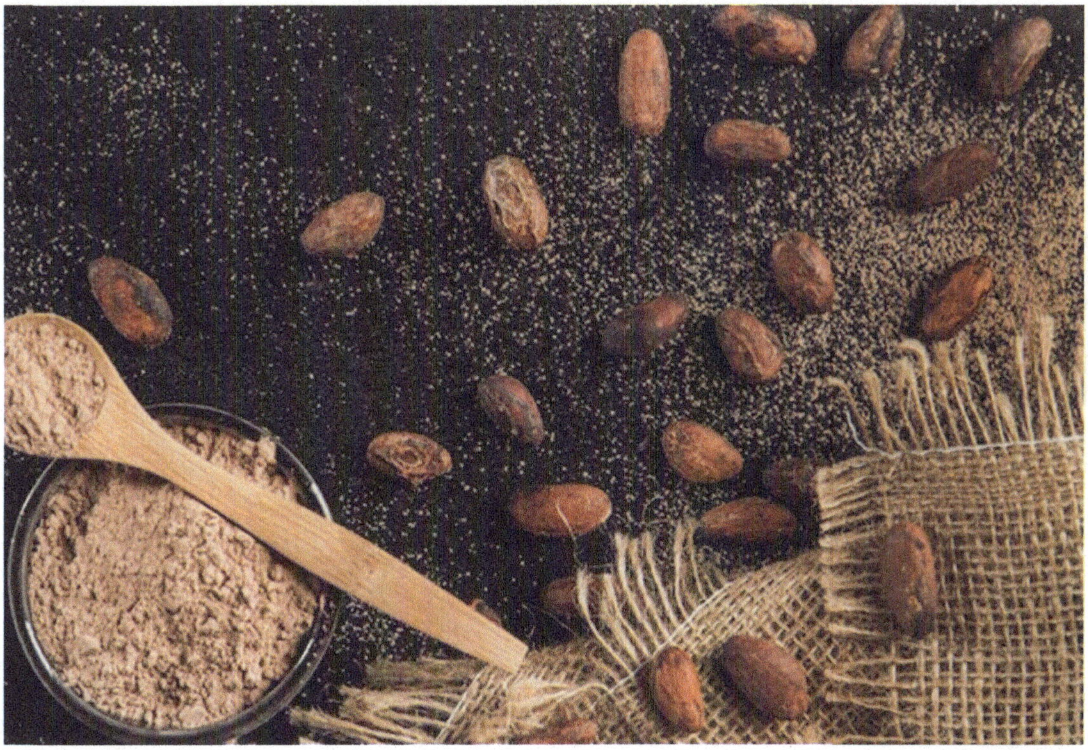

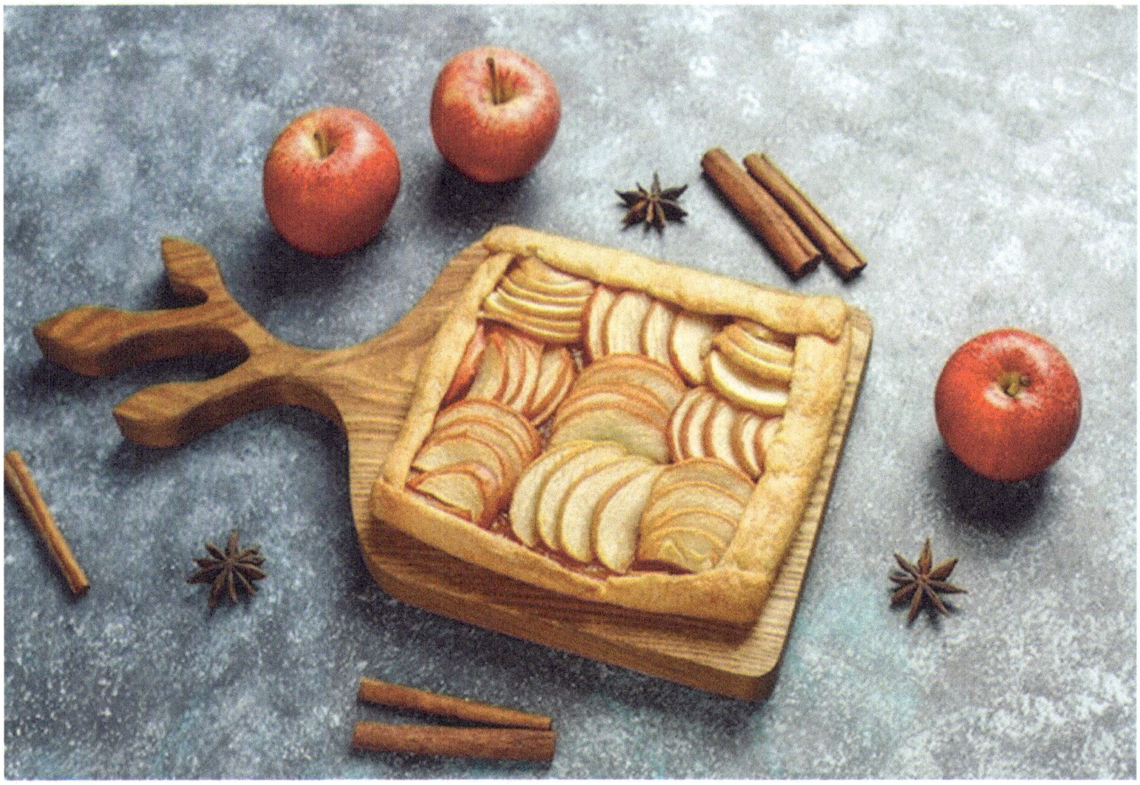

13. Baked Cinnamon Apples

Prep.Time: 10 min

Cook Time: 25 min

Serving: 4

Beverage pairing: Herbal Tea

Ingredients:

- 4 medium-sized apples, cored and sliced
- 1 tablespoon melted coconut oil
- 1 teaspoon ground cinnamon
- 1/4 teaspoon nutmeg
- 1/4 cup chopped walnuts (optional)
- 1 tablespoon sugar-free sweetener (erythritol or stevia)

Preparation:

1. Preheat the oven to 375°F (190°C).
2. In a bowl, toss the apple slices with melted coconut oil, ground cinnamon, nutmeg, chopped walnuts (if using), and sugar-free sweetener.
3. Transfer the coated apples to a baking dish.
4. Bake for 20-25 minutes or until the apples are tender.
5. Serve warm, optionally topped with a dollop of sugar-free whipped cream.

Nutrient Facts (per serving):

- Calories: 120
- Carbohydrates: 18g
- Fat: 6g
- Protein: 1g

14. Chia Seed Coconut Macaroons

Prep.Time: 15 min

Cook Time: 18 min

Serving: 12

Beverage pairing: Herbal Tea

Ingredients:

- 2 cups shredded coconut (unsweetened)
- 1/4 cup coconut flour
- 1/4 cup chia seeds
- 1/3 cup melted coconut oil
- 1/4 cup sugar-free sweetener (erythritol or stevia)
- 1 teaspoon vanilla extract
- A pinch of salt

Preparation:

1. Preheat the oven to 325°F (163°C) and line a baking sheet with parchment paper.
2. In a bowl, combine shredded coconut, coconut flour, chia seeds, melted coconut oil, sugar-free sweetener, vanilla extract, and a pinch of salt. Mix well.
3. Using a cookie scoop or your hands, form small mounds of the mixture and place them on the prepared baking sheet.
4. Bake for 15-18 minutes or until the edges are golden brown.
5. Allow the macaroons to cool on the baking sheet for 5 minutes before transferring them to a wire rack to cool completely.

Nutrient Facts (per macaroon - makes approximately 12):

- Calories: 90
- Carbohydrates: 4g
- Fat: 8g
- Protein: 1g

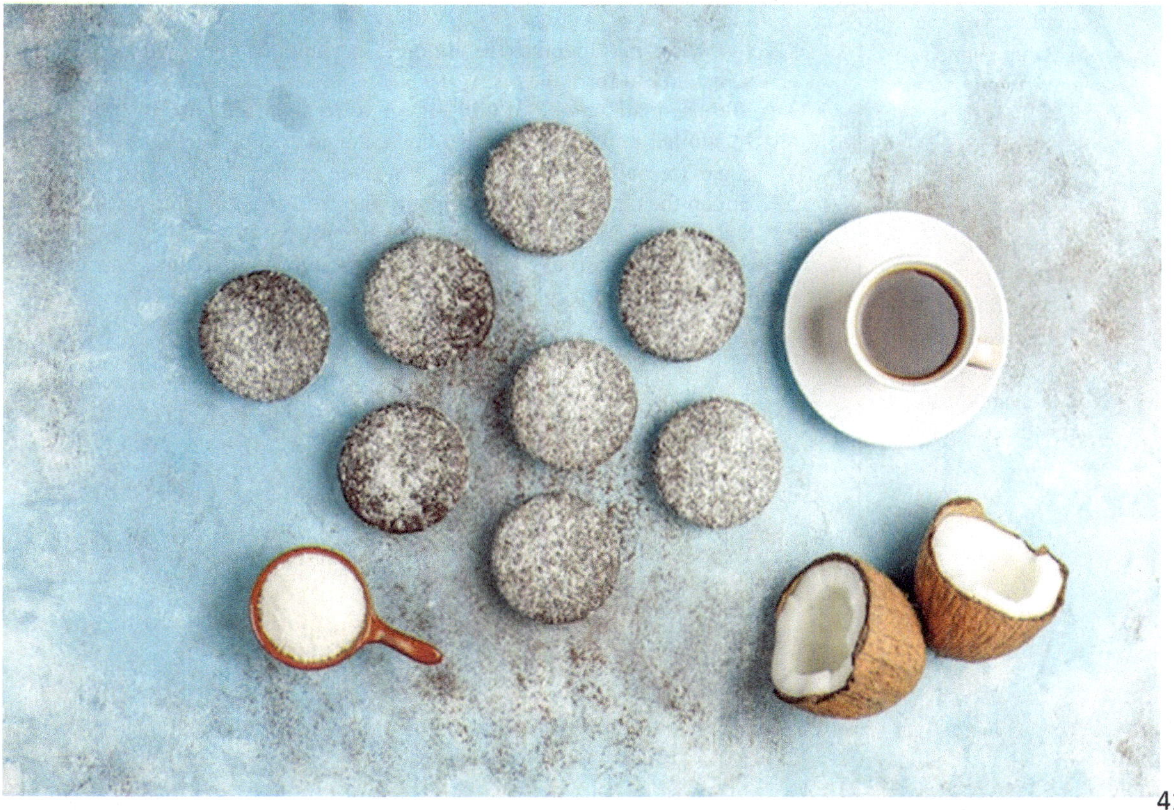

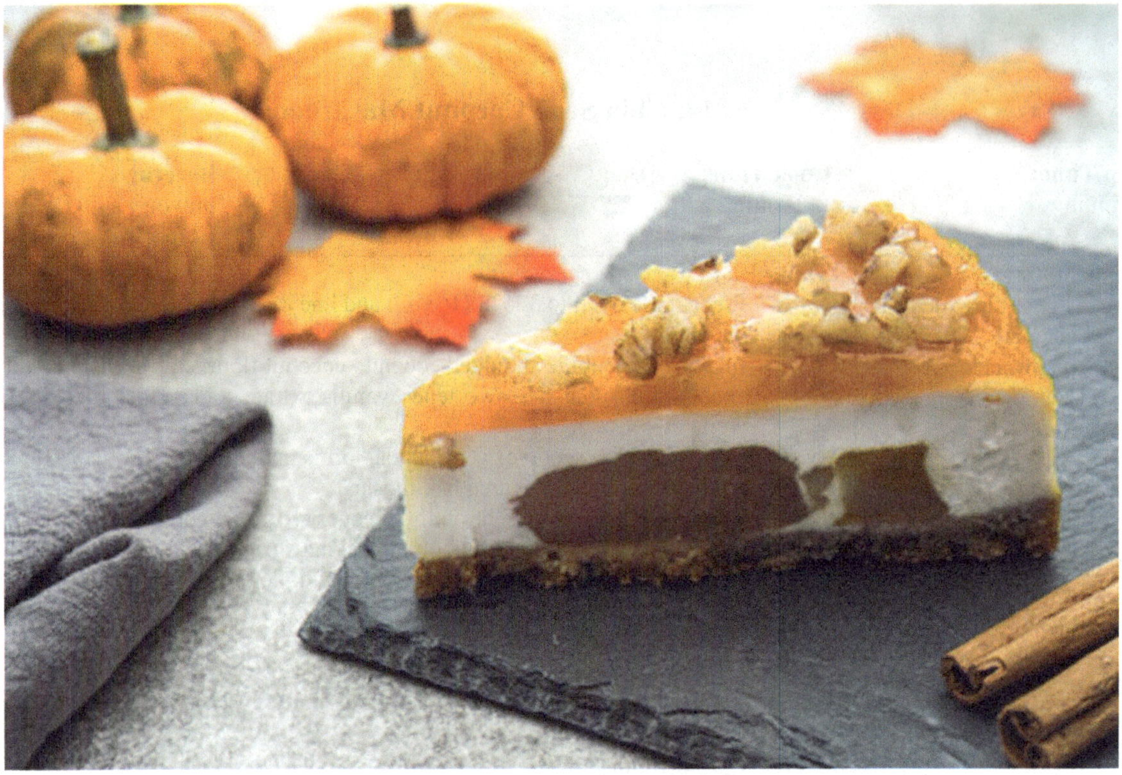

15. Low-Carb Pumpkin Cheesecake Bites

Prep.Time: 15 min

Cook Time: 18 min

Serving: 24

Beverage pairing: Coffee

Ingredients:

- 8 oz cream cheese (softened)
- 1/2 cup canned pumpkin puree
- 1/4 cup sugar-free sweetener (erythritol or stevia)
- 1 teaspoon pumpkin spice
- 1 cup almond flour
- 1/4 cup melted butter
- 1 tablespoon sugar-free sweetener

Preparation:

1. Preheat the oven to 325°F (163°C) and line a mini muffin tin with paper liners.
2. In a bowl, mix together the almond flour, melted butter, and sugar-free sweetener to form the crust.
3. Press a small amount of the crust mixture into each muffin cup.
4. In another bowl, beat together the softened cream cheese, pumpkin puree, sugar-free sweetener, and pumpkin spice until smooth.
5. Spoon the cheesecake mixture onto the crust in each muffin cup.
6. Bake for 15-18 minutes or until the cheesecake is set.
7. Allow the cheesecake bites to cool in the muffin tin before transferring them to the refrigerator to chill.

Nutrient Facts (per cheesecake bite - makes approximately 24):

- Calories: 80
- Carbohydrates: 2g
- Fat: 7g
- Protein: 2g

16. Vanilla Almond Protein Bites

Prep.Time:	Cook Time:	Serving:	Beverage pairing:
10 min	30 min	12	Herbal Tea

Ingredients:

- 1 cup almond flour
- 1/4 cup vanilla protein powder
- 1/4 cup almond butter
- 1/4 cup melted coconut oil
- 1 teaspoon vanilla extract
- 1 tablespoon sugar-free sweetener (erythritol or stevia)
- A pinch of salt
- Sliced almonds for coating (optional)

Preparation:

1. In a bowl, combine almond flour, vanilla protein powder, almond butter, melted coconut oil, vanilla extract, sugar-free sweetener, and a pinch of salt. Mix until well combined.
2. Form small balls from the mixture. Optionally, roll the balls in sliced almonds for coating.
3. Refrigerate for at least 30 minutes before serving.

Nutrient Facts (per protein bite - makes approximately 12):

- Calories: 90
- Carbohydrates: 3g
- Fat: 7g
- Protein: 3g

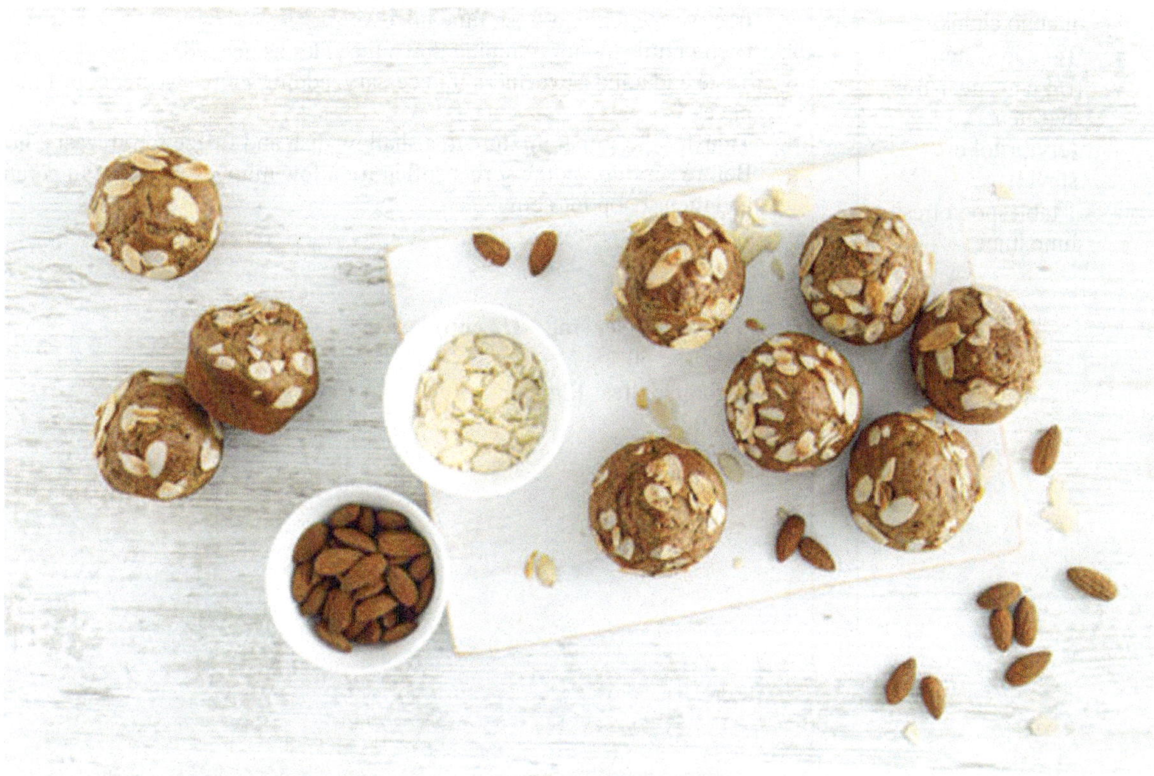

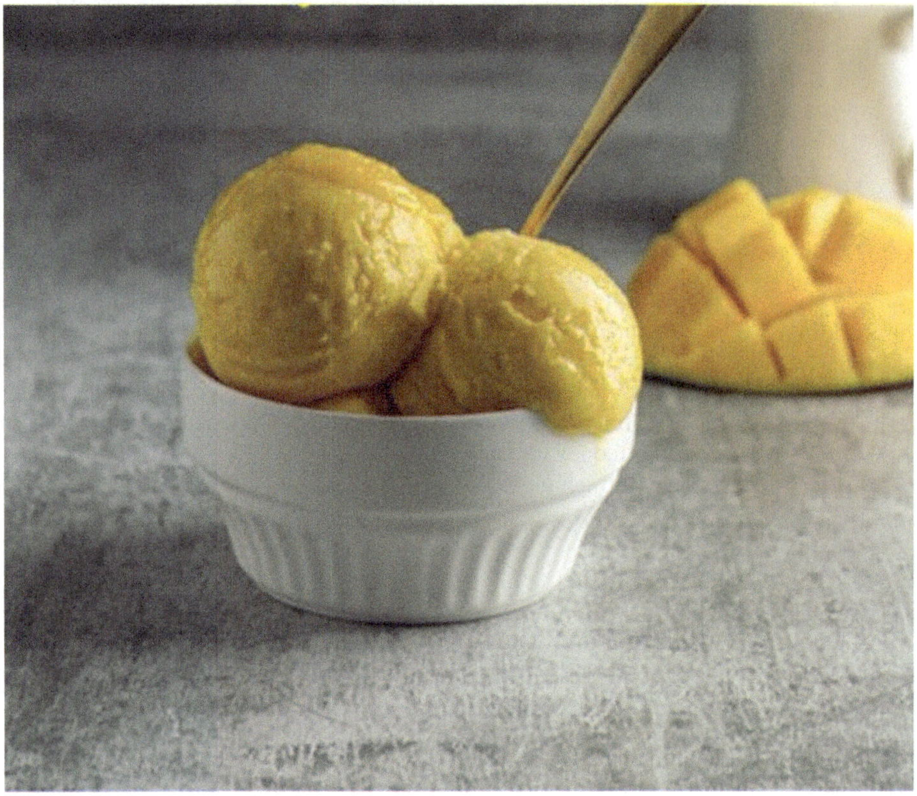

17. Sugar-Free Mango Sorbet

Prep.Time:	Cook Time:	Serving:	Beverage pairing:
10 min	0 min	6	Herbal Tea

Ingredients:

- 2 cups frozen mango chunks
- 1/4 cup water
- 1/4 cup sugar-free sweetener (erythritol or stevia)
- 1 tablespoon fresh lime juice

Preparation:

1. In a blender or food processor, combine frozen mango chunks, water, sugar-free sweetener, and fresh lime juice.
2. Blend until smooth, scraping down the sides as needed.
3. Taste and adjust sweetness if necessary, adding more sweetener or lime juice.
4. Transfer the sorbet mixture to a shallow dish and freeze for at least 2 hours.
5. Before serving, let the sorbet soften for a few minutes at room temperature and then scoop into bowls.

Nutrient Facts (per serving - 1/2 cup):

- Calories: 50
- Carbohydrates: 12g
- Fat: 0g
- Protein: 1g

18. Cranberry Walnut Energy Bites

Prep.Time:	Cook Time:	Serving:	Beverage pairing:
15 min	30 min	12	Green Tea

Ingredients:

- 1 cup rolled oats
- 1/2 cup dried cranberries (unsweetened)
- 1/2 cup chopped walnuts
- 1/4 cup almond butter
- 1/4 cup honey or sugar-free sweetener
- 1 teaspoon vanilla extract
- A pinch of salt

Preparation:

1. In a food processor, combine rolled oats, dried cranberries, chopped walnuts, almond butter, honey or sugar-free sweetener, vanilla extract, and a pinch of salt.
2. Pulse until the mixture comes together and forms a sticky dough.
3. Roll the dough into bite-sized balls and place them on a parchment-lined tray.
4. Refrigerate for at least 30 minutes before serving.

Nutrient Facts (per energy bite - makes approximately 12):

- Calories: 120
- Carbohydrates: 14g
- Fat: 6g
- Protein: 3g

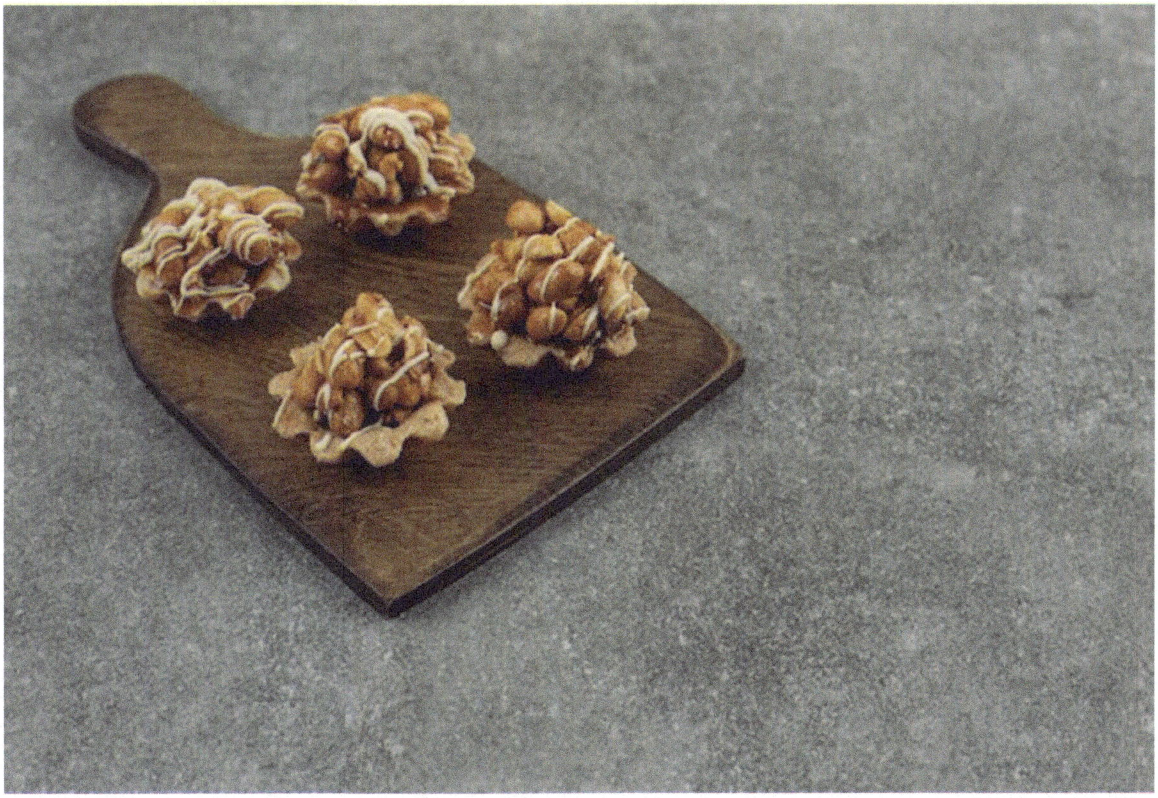

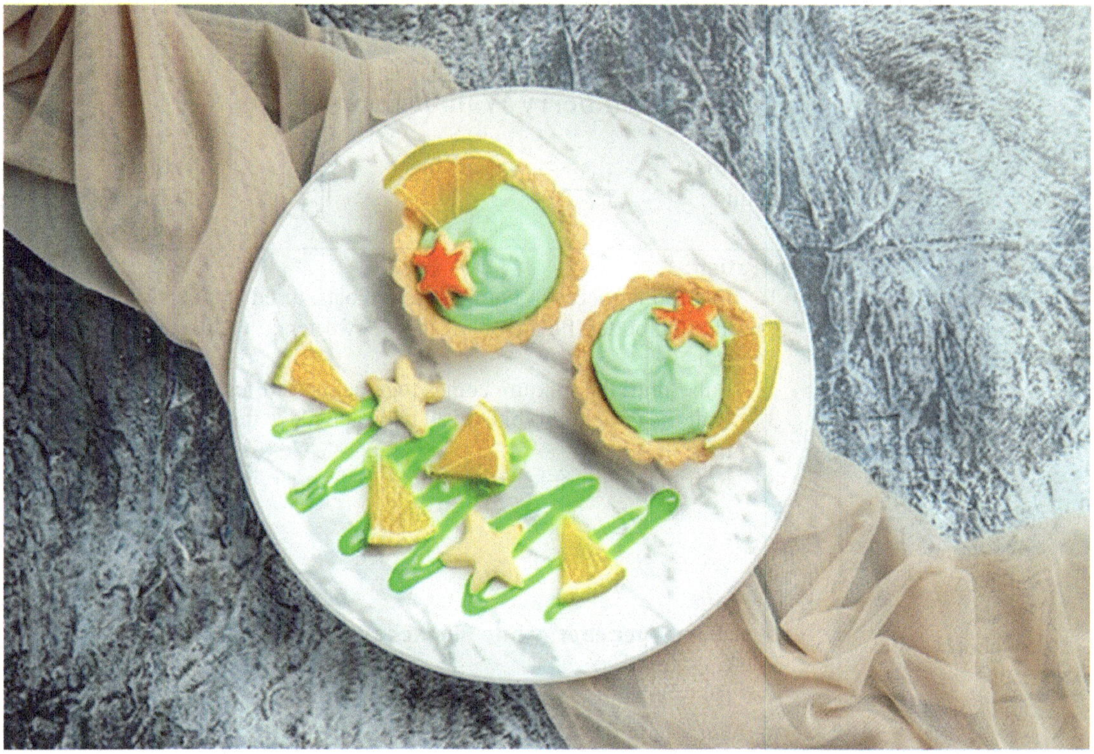

19. Avocado Lime Cheesecake Cups

Prep.Time: 15 min

Cook Time: 20 min

Serving: 12

Beverage pairing: Mint Tea

Ingredients:

- 1 ripe avocado
- 8 oz cream cheese (softened)
- 1/4 cup lime juice
- 1/4 cup sugar-free sweetener (erythritol or stevia)
- 1 teaspoon lime zest
- 1 cup almond flour
- 1/4 cup melted butter
- 1 tablespoon sugar-free sweetener

Preparation:

1. Preheat the oven to 325°F (163°C) and line a muffin tin with paper liners.
2. In a food processor, blend together the avocado, softened cream cheese, lime juice, sugar-free sweetener, and lime zest until smooth.
3. In a bowl, mix almond flour, melted butter, and sugar-free sweetener to form the crust.
4. Press a small amount of the crust mixture into each muffin cup.
5. Spoon the avocado-lime cheesecake mixture onto the crust in each muffin cup.
6. Bake for 15-18 minutes or until the cheesecake is set.
7. Allow the cheesecake cups to cool in the muffin tin before transferring them to the refrigerator to chill.

Nutrient Facts (per cheesecake cup - makes approximately 12):

- Calories: 120
- Carbohydrates: 4g
- Fat: 11g
- Protein: 3g

20. Berry and Greek Yogurt Popsicles

Prep.Time:	Cook Time:	Serving:	Beverage pairing:
10 min	0 min	6	Hibiscus Tea

Ingredients:

- 1 cup mixed berries (strawberries, blueberries, raspberries)
- 1 cup Greek yogurt (unsweetened)
- 1/4 cup sugar-free sweetener (erythritol or stevia)
- 1 teaspoon vanilla extract

Preparation:

1. In a blender, puree the mixed berries until smooth.
2. In a bowl, mix Greek yogurt, sugar-free sweetener, and vanilla extract.
3. Layer the berry puree and Greek yogurt mixture into popsicle molds.
4. Insert popsicle sticks and freeze for at least 4 hours or until solid.

Nutrient Facts (per popsicle - makes approximately 6):

- Calories: 50
- Carbohydrates: 7g
- Fat: 1g
- Protein: 4g

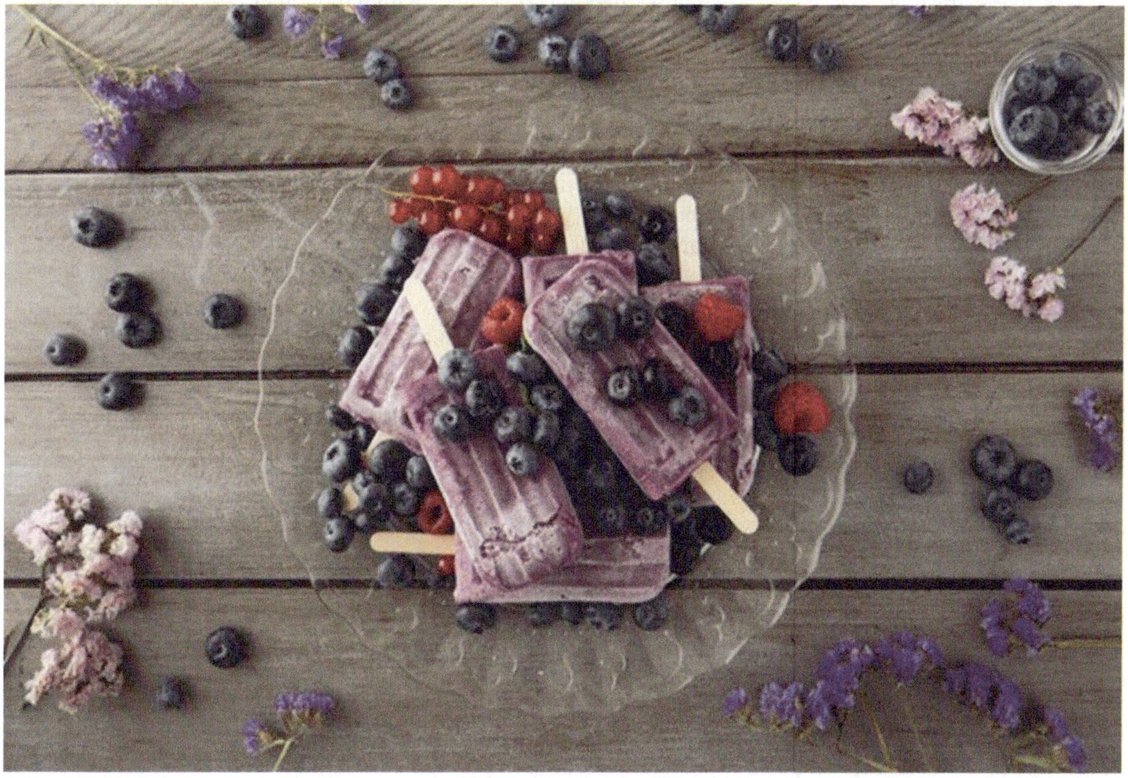

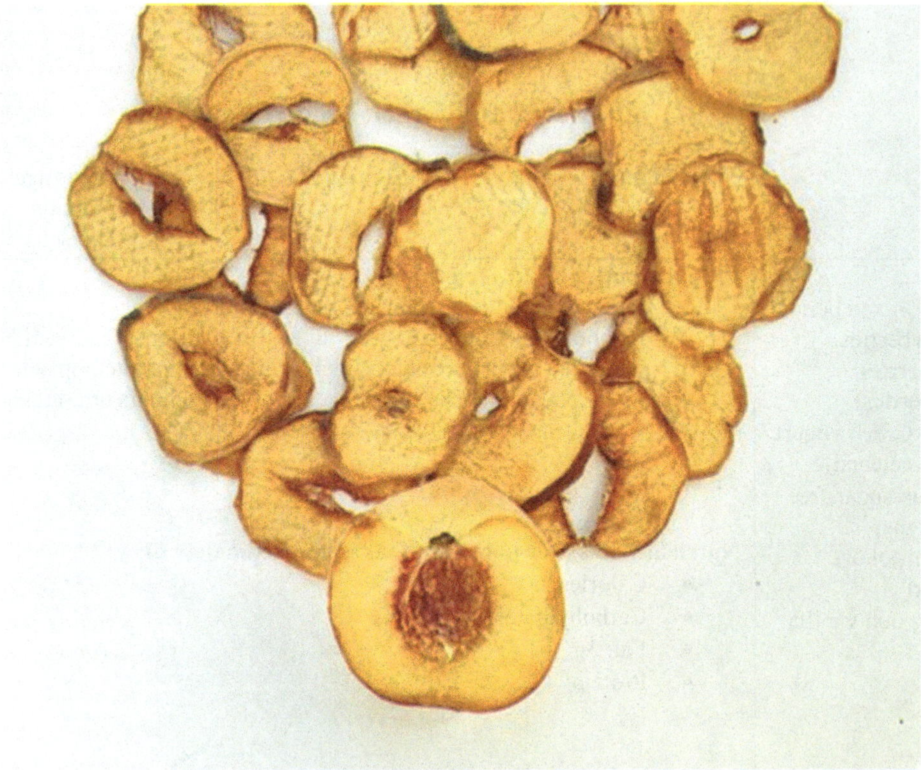

21. Peach Almond Crisp

Prep.Time: 15 min

Cook Time: 30 min

Serving: 6

Beverage pairing: Cinnamon Tea

Ingredients:

- 4 cups sliced peaches (fresh or frozen)
- 2 tablespoons lemon juice
- 2 tablespoons sugar-free sweetener (erythritol or stevia)
- 1 teaspoon vanilla extract
- 1 cup almond flour
- 1/2 cup sliced almonds
- 1/4 cup melted butter
- 1/4 cup sugar-free sweetener
- 1/2 teaspoon ground cinnamon

Preparation:

1. Preheat the oven to 350°F (175°C).
2. In a bowl, toss sliced peaches with lemon juice, sugar-free sweetener, and vanilla extract. Transfer to a baking dish.
3. In another bowl, combine almond flour, sliced almonds, melted butter, sugar-free sweetener, ground cinnamon, and a pinch of salt to make the crisp topping.
4. Sprinkle the crisp topping over the peach filling.
5. Bake for 25-30 minutes or until the topping is golden brown and the peaches are bubbly.
6. Allow the peach almond crisp to cool slightly before serving.

Nutrient Facts (per serving - serves approximately 6):

- Calories: 250
- Carbohydrates: 16g
- Fat: 20g
- Protein: 5g

22. No-Sugar Added Poached Pears

Prep.Time:	Cook Time:	Serving:	Beverage pairing:
10 min	20 min	4	Chamomile Tea

Ingredients:

- 4 ripe but firm pears, peeled and cored
- 4 cups water
- 1 cinnamon stick
- 2-3 whole cloves
- 1 teaspoon vanilla extract
- 1 tablespoon lemon juice
- Sugar-free sweetener to taste (erythritol or stevia)

Preparation:

1. In a pot, combine water, cinnamon stick, whole cloves, vanilla extract, lemon juice, and sugar-free sweetener.
2. Bring the liquid to a simmer over medium heat.
3. Add the peeled and cored pears to the simmering liquid.
4. Poach the pears for 20-25 minutes or until they are tender but not mushy.
5. Remove the pears from the liquid and allow them to cool.
6. Optionally, reduce the poaching liquid until it thickens and drizzle it over the pears before serving.

Nutrient Facts (per pear - serves 4):

- Calories: 100
- Carbohydrates: 25g
- Fat: 0g
- Protein: 1g

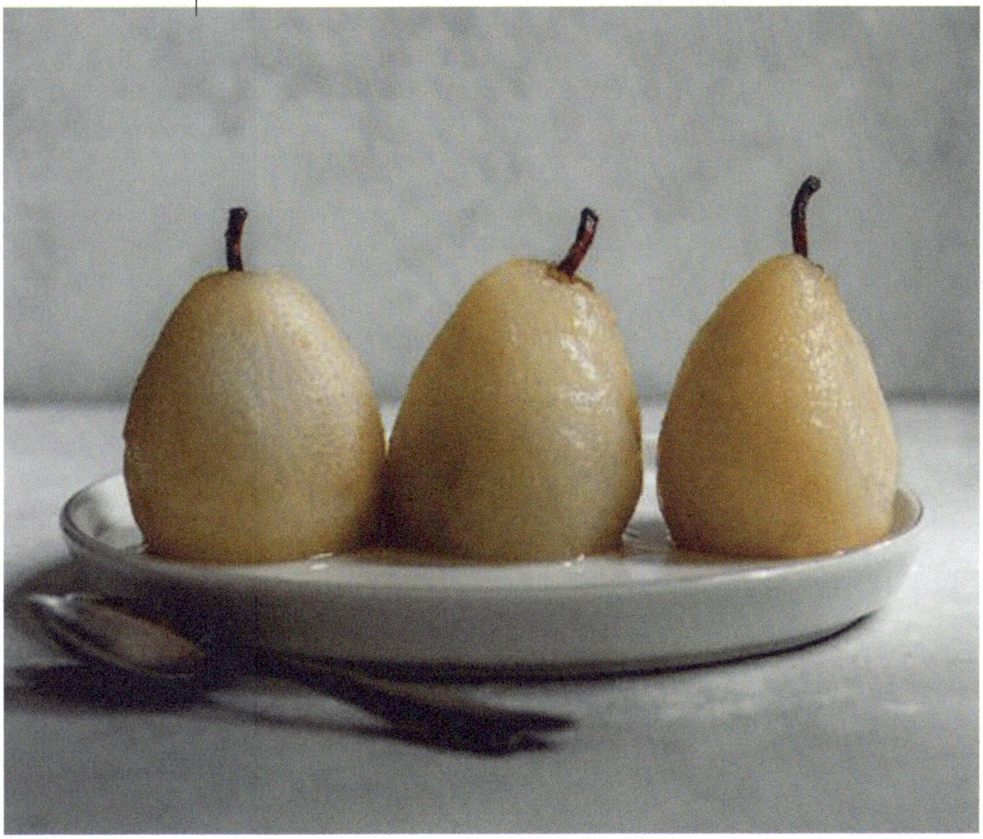

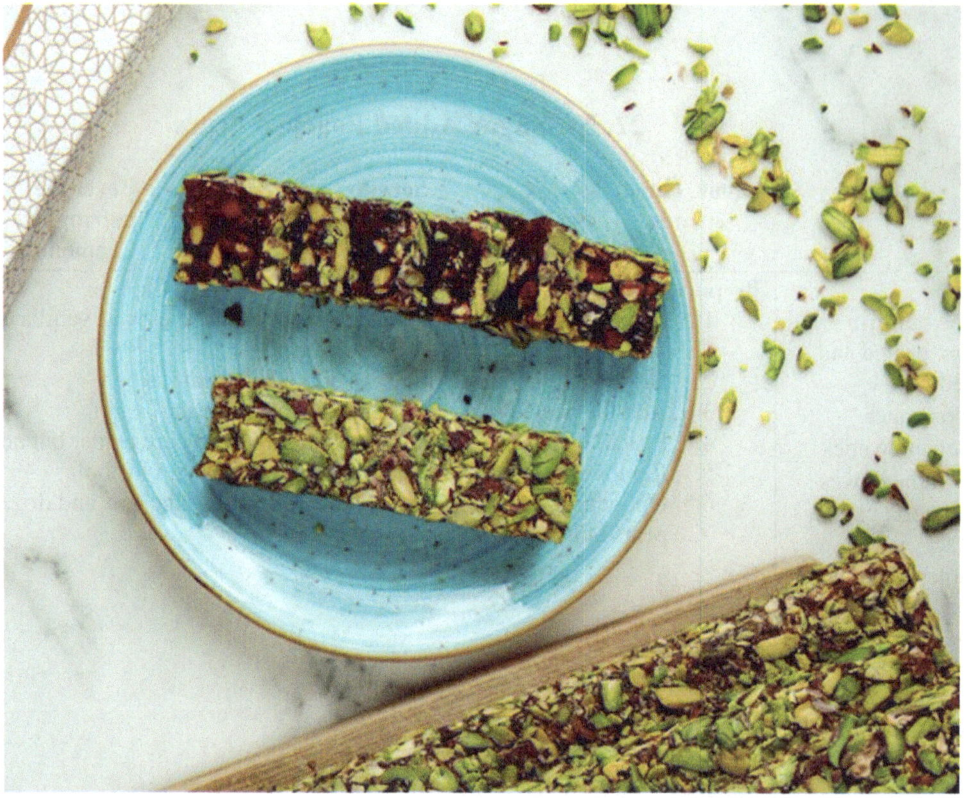

23. Pistachio Dark Chocolate Bark

Prep.Time:	Cook Time:	Serving:	Beverage pairing:
10 min	60 min	8	Black Tea

Ingredients:

- 1 cup dark chocolate chips (sugar-free or at least 70% cocoa)
- 1/2 cup shelled pistachios, chopped
- 1/4 cup unsweetened shredded coconut
- A pinch of sea salt

Preparation:

1. Line a tray with parchment paper.
2. Melt the dark chocolate chips in a microwave-safe bowl in 30-second intervals, stirring between each interval until smooth.
3. Spread the melted chocolate onto the parchment paper.
4. Sprinkle chopped pistachios, shredded coconut, and a pinch of sea salt over the melted chocolate.
5. Refrigerate for at least 1 hour or until the chocolate is set.
6. Break the chocolate bark into pieces before serving.

Nutrient Facts (per serving - makes approximately 8):

- Calories: 120
- Carbohydrates: 10g
- Fat: 8g
- Protein: 2g

24. Sugar-Free Coconut Rice Pudding

Prep.Time:	**Cook Time:**	**Serving:**	**Beverage pairing:**
5 min	30 min	4	Herbal Tea

Ingredients:

- 1 cup Arborio rice
- 2 cups unsweetened coconut milk
- 2 cups water
- 1/4 cup sugar-free sweetener (erythritol or stevia)
- 1/2 teaspoon vanilla extract
- A pinch of salt
- Unsweetened shredded coconut for garnish

Preparation:

1. In a pot, combine Arborio rice, coconut milk, water, sugar-free sweetener, vanilla extract, and a pinch of salt.
2. Bring the mixture to a boil, then reduce the heat to low and simmer, stirring occasionally, for 25-30 minutes or until the rice is tender.
3. Remove the pot from heat and let the rice pudding cool.
4. Refrigerate for at least 2 hours before serving.
5. Garnish with unsweetened shredded coconut before serving.

Nutrient Facts (per serving - serves approximately 4):

- Calories: 200
- Carbohydrates: 30g
- Fat: 7g
- Protein: 2g

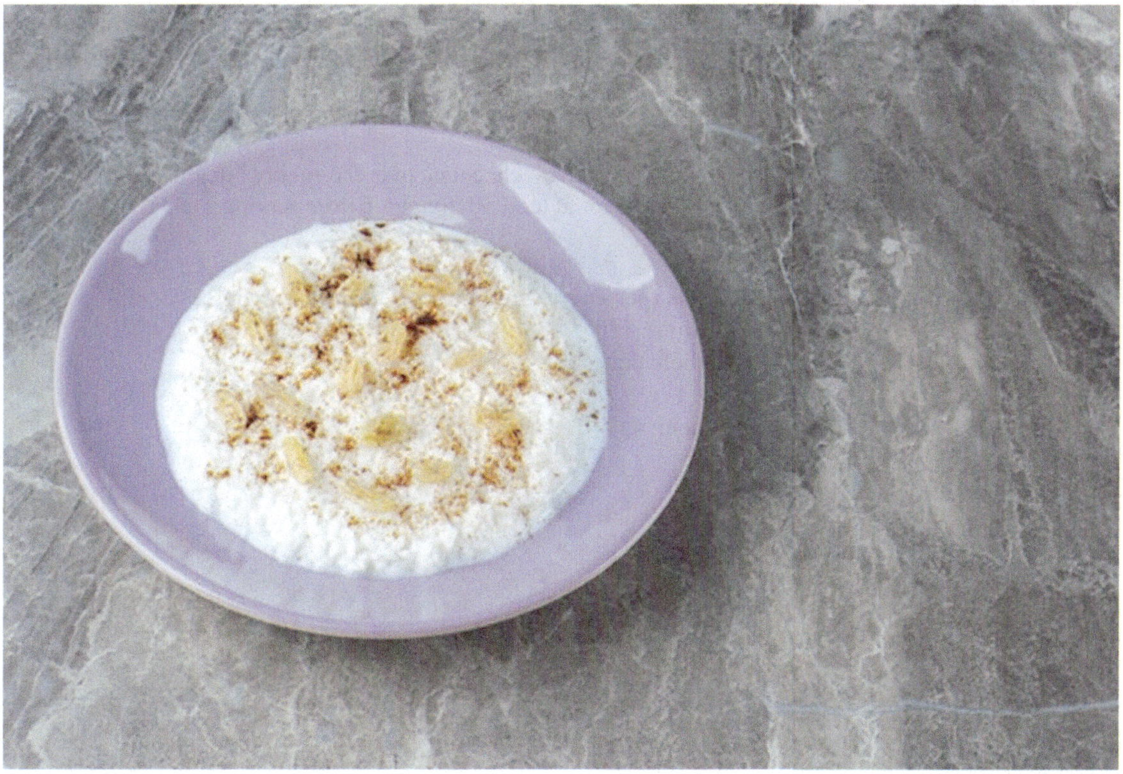

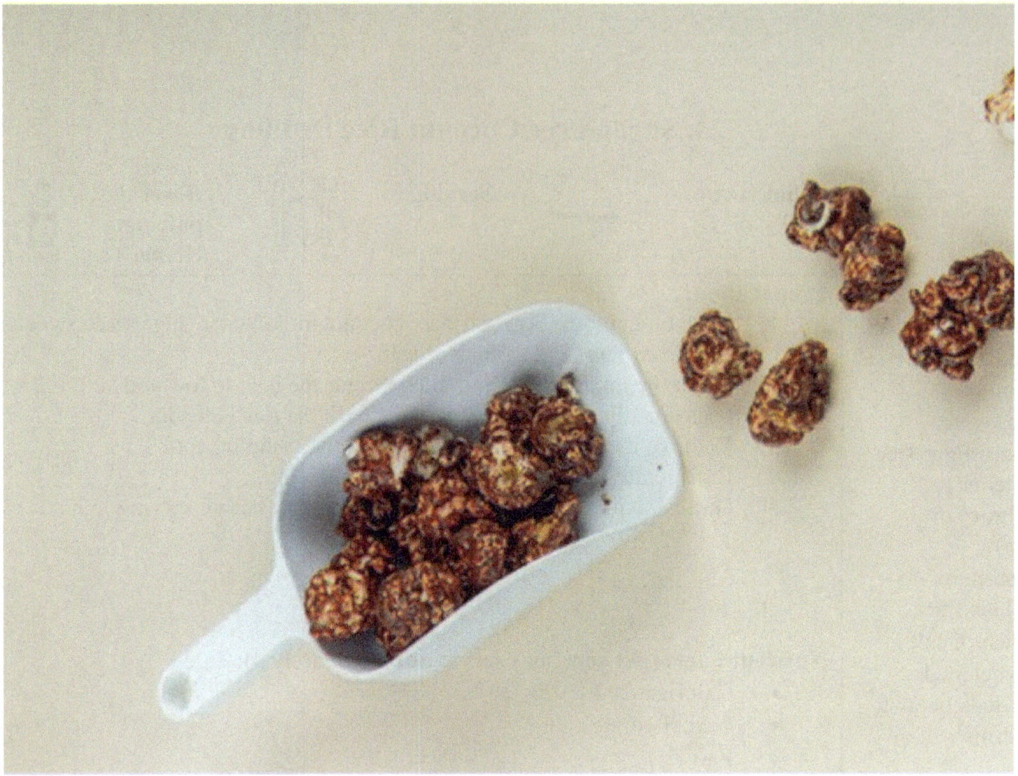

25. Almond Joy Energy Bites

Prep.Time: 15 min	Cook Time: 30 min	Serving: 12	Beverage pairing: Iced Coffee

Ingredients:

- 1 cup almonds
- 1 cup shredded coconut (unsweetened)
- 1/4 cup almond butter
- 1/4 cup sugar-free sweetener (erythritol or stevia)
- 1 teaspoon vanilla extract
- A pinch of salt
- 1/4 cup dark chocolate chips (sugar-free or at least 70% cocoa), melted

Preparation:

1. In a food processor, blend almonds until finely chopped.
2. Add shredded coconut, almond butter, sugar-free sweetener, vanilla extract, and a pinch of salt to the food processor. Blend until the mixture sticks together.
3. Roll the mixture into bite-sized balls and place them on a parchment-lined tray.
4. Drizzle melted dark chocolate over the energy bites.
5. Refrigerate for at least 30 minutes before serving.

Nutrient Facts (per energy bite - makes approximately 12):

- Calories: 150
- Carbohydrates: 8g
- Fat: 12g
- Protein: 4g

26. Baked Cinnamon Bananas

Prep.Time: 10 min

Cook Time: 20 min

Serving: 4

Beverage pairing: Chamomile Tea

Ingredients:

- 4 ripe but firm bananas, peeled and sliced
- 2 tablespoons melted coconut oil
- 1 teaspoon ground cinnamon
- 1 tablespoon sugar-free sweetener (erythritol or stevia)

Preparation:

1. Preheat the oven to 350°F (175°C) and line a baking sheet with parchment paper.
2. In a bowl, toss the banana slices with melted coconut oil, ground cinnamon, and sugar-free sweetener.
3. Arrange the banana slices on the prepared baking sheet.
4. Bake for 15-20 minutes or until the bananas are soft and caramelized.
5. Serve warm, optionally topped with a sprinkle of extra cinnamon.

Nutrient Facts (per serving - serves approximately 4):

- Calories: 120
- Carbohydrates: 22g
- Fat: 5g
- Protein: 1g

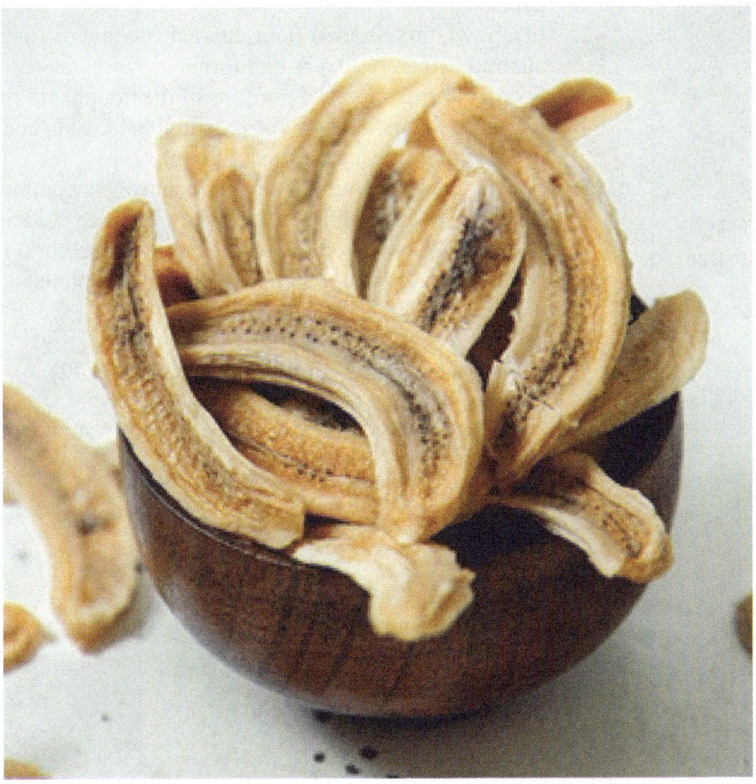

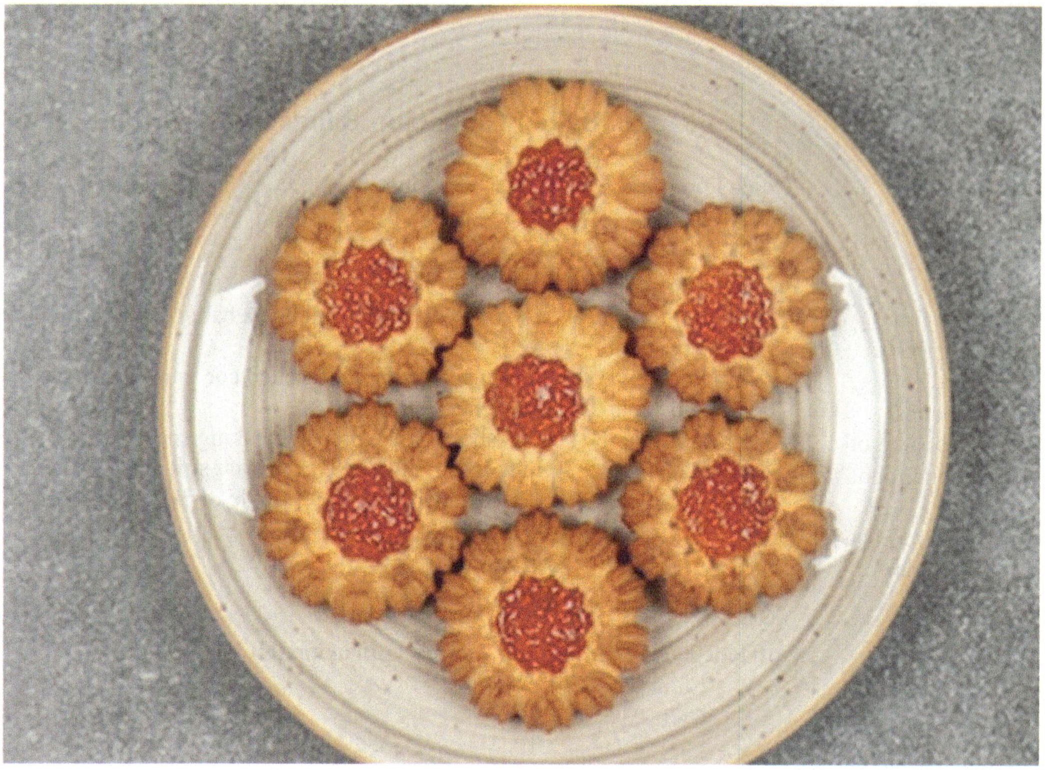

27. Raspberry Almond Thumbprint Cookies

Prep.Time: 15 min

Cook Time: 12 min

Serving: 12

Beverage pairing: Earl Grey Tea

Ingredients:

- 1 cup almond flour
- 1/4 cup melted coconut oil
- 1/4 cup sugar-free sweetener (erythritol or stevia)
- 1/2 teaspoon almond extract
- 1/4 cup sugar-free raspberry jam

Preparation:

1. Preheat the oven to 350°F (175°C) and line a baking sheet with parchment paper.
2. In a bowl, mix almond flour, melted coconut oil, sugar-free sweetener, and almond extract until a dough forms.
3. Scoop tablespoon-sized portions of the dough and roll them into balls.
4. Place the dough balls on the prepared baking sheet and make an indentation in the center of each with your thumb.
5. Spoon a small amount of sugar-free raspberry jam into each indentation.
6. Bake for 10-12 minutes or until the edges are golden brown.
7. Allow the cookies to cool on the baking sheet for 5 minutes before transferring them to a wire rack to cool completely.

Nutrient Facts (per cookie - makes approximately 12):

- Calories: 80
- Carbohydrates: 5g
- Fat: 7g
- Protein: 2g

28. Sugar-Free Lemon Sorbet

Prep.Time:	Cook Time:	Serving:	Beverage pairing:
10 min	0 min	6	Iced Tea

Ingredients:

- 2 cups water
- 1 cup fresh lemon juice
- Zest of 2 lemons
- 1/2 cup sugar-free sweetener (erythritol or stevia)
- 1/4 teaspoon lemon extract (optional)

Preparation:

1. In a bowl, combine water, fresh lemon juice, lemon zest, sugar-free sweetener, and lemon extract (if using). Stir until the sweetener is dissolved.
2. Pour the mixture into an ice cream maker and churn according to the manufacturer's instructions.
3. Transfer the sorbet to a shallow dish and freeze for at least 2 hours.
4. Before serving, let the sorbet soften for a few minutes at room temperature and then scoop into bowls.

Nutrient Facts (per serving - 1/2 cup):

- Calories: 20
- Carbohydrates: 5g
- Fat: 0g
- Protein: 0g

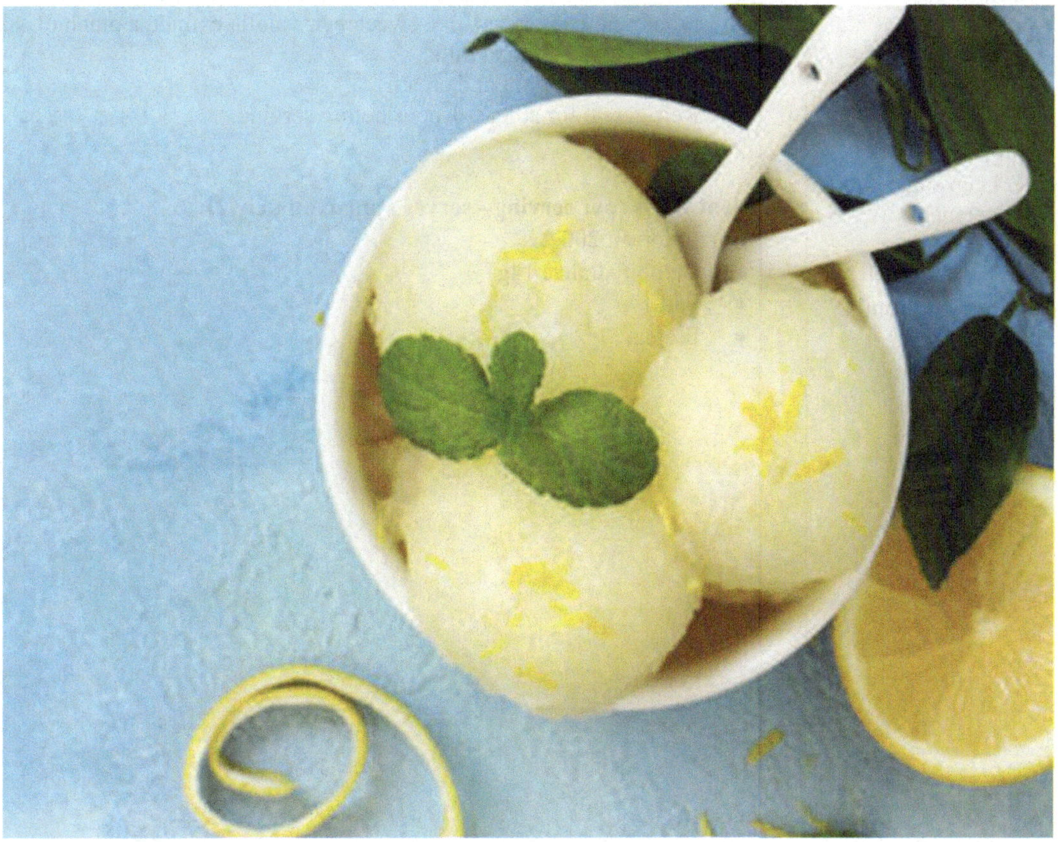

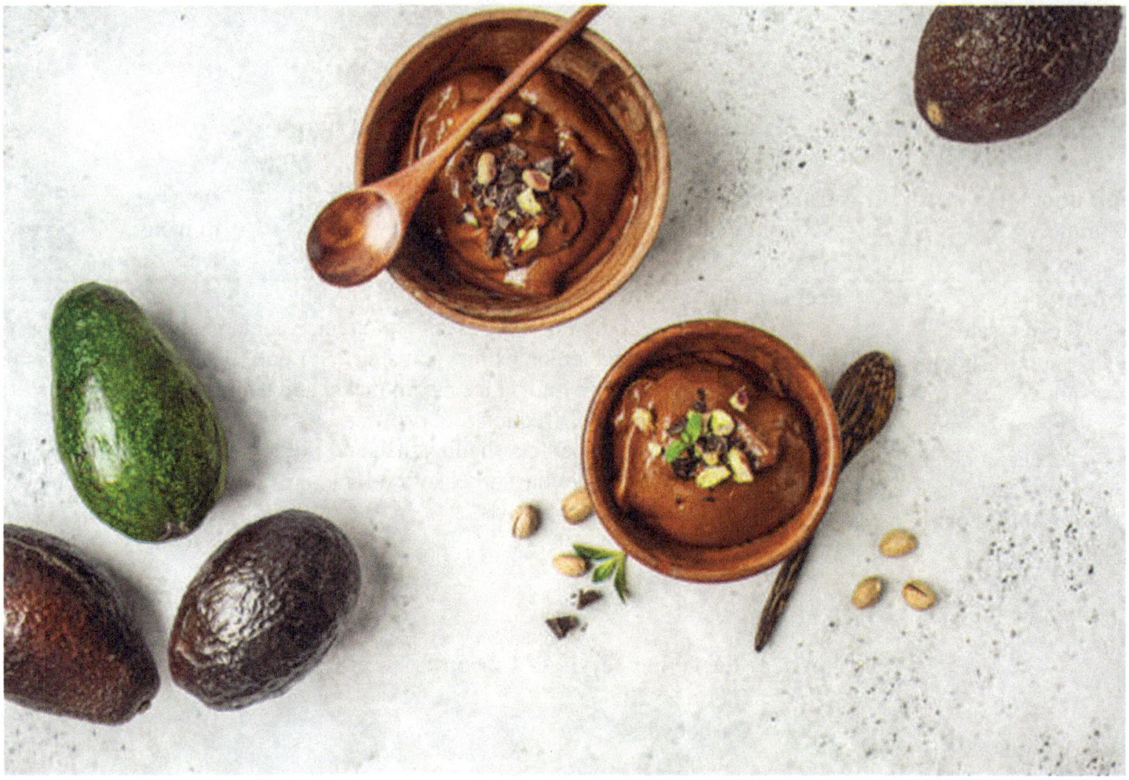

29. Chocolate Avocado Protein Pudding

Prep.Time:	Cook Time:	Serving:	Beverage pairing:
10 min	60 min	2	Black Coffee

Ingredients:

- 2 ripe avocados
- 1/4 cup cocoa powder (unsweetened)
- 1/4 cup chocolate protein powder
- 1/4 cup sugar-free sweetener (erythritol or stevia)
- 1 teaspoon vanilla extract
- A pinch of salt
- 1/2 cup unsweetened almond milk

Preparation:

1. In a blender or food processor, combine avocados, cocoa powder, chocolate protein powder, sugar-free sweetener, vanilla extract, a pinch of salt, and unsweetened almond milk.
2. Blend until smooth and creamy.
3. Refrigerate for at least 1 hour before serving.

Nutrient Facts (per serving - serves approximately 2):

- Calories: 200
- Carbohydrates: 14g
- Fat: 14g
- Protein: 7g

30. Walnut and Date Protein Balls

Prep.Time:	Cook Time:	Serving:	Beverage pairing:
15 min	30 min	12	Herbal Tea

Ingredients:

- 1 cup walnuts
- 1 cup pitted dates
- 1/4 cup vanilla protein powder
- 1/4 cup unsweetened shredded coconut
- 1 teaspoon vanilla extract
- A pinch of salt

Preparation:

1. In a food processor, blend walnuts, pitted dates, vanilla protein powder, shredded coconut, vanilla extract, and a pinch of salt until the mixture forms a sticky dough.
2. Scoop out tablespoon-sized portions of the mixture and roll them into balls.
3. Refrigerate for at least 30 minutes before serving.

Nutrient Facts (per protein ball - makes approximately 12):

- Calories: 100
- Carbohydrates: 10g
- Fat: 6g
- Protein: 3g

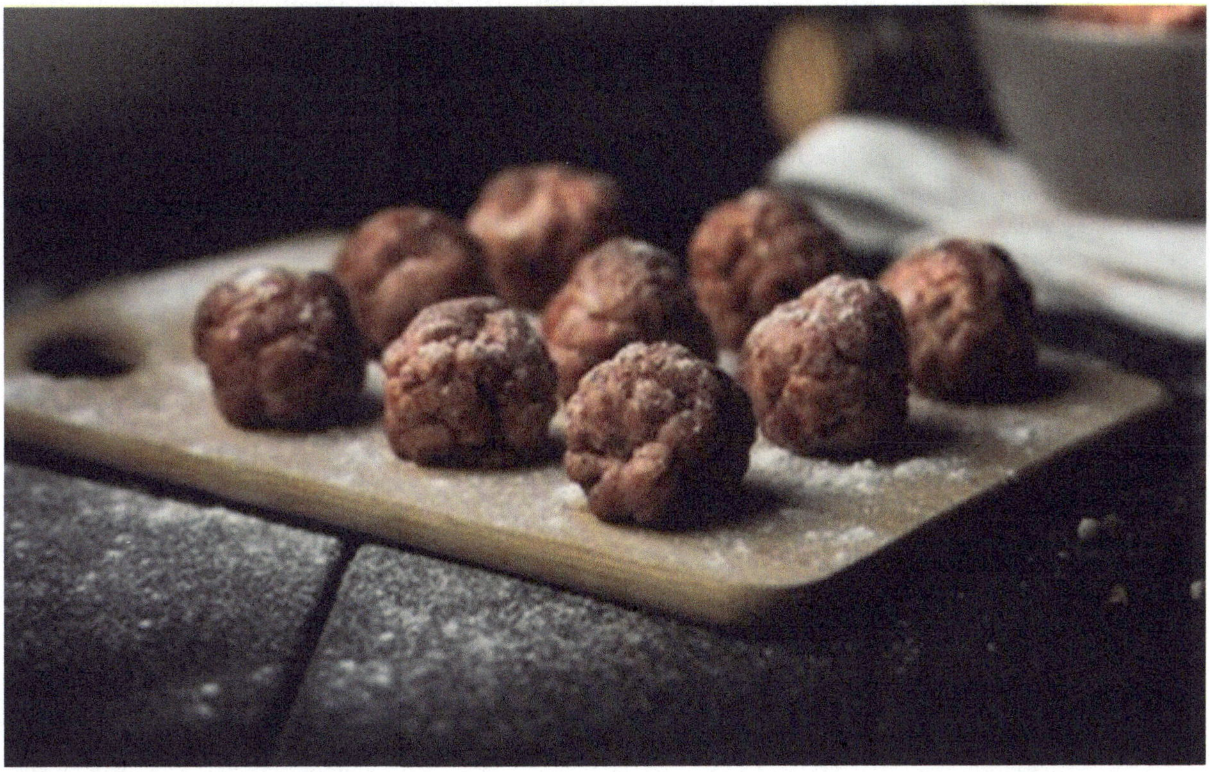

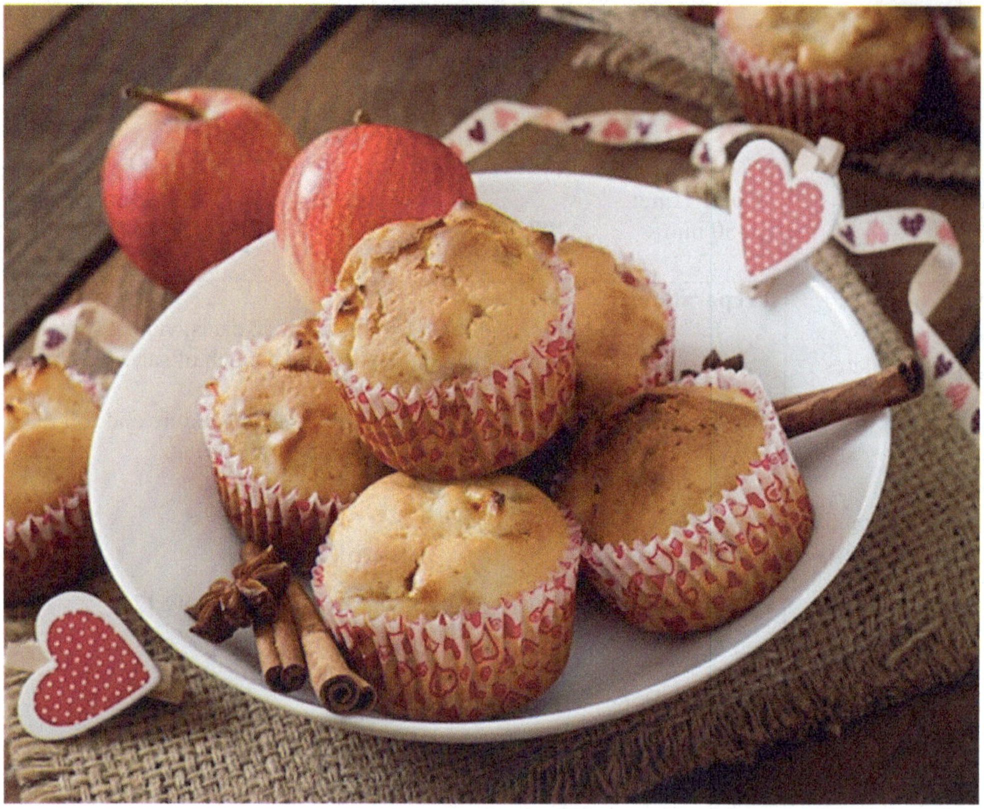

31. Sugar-Free Apple Cinnamon Muffins

Prep.Time:	Cook Time:	Serving:	Beverage pairing:
15 min	25 min	12	Black Coffee

Ingredients:

- 2 cups almond flour
- 1/4 cup coconut flour
- 1 teaspoon baking powder
- 1/2 teaspoon baking soda
- 1 teaspoon ground cinnamon
- 1/4 cup melted coconut oil
- 1/4 cup unsweetened applesauce
- 3 large eggs
- 1/4 cup sugar-free sweetener (erythritol or stevia)
- 1 teaspoon vanilla extract
- 1 cup grated apple (peeled)

Preparation:

1. Preheat the oven to 350°F (175°C) and line a muffin tin with paper liners.
2. In a bowl, whisk together almond flour, coconut flour, baking powder, baking soda, and ground cinnamon.
3. In another bowl, combine melted coconut oil, unsweetened applesauce, eggs, sugar-free sweetener, and vanilla extract. Mix well.
4. Add the wet ingredients to the dry ingredients and stir until just combined.
5. Fold in the grated apple.
6. Spoon the batter into the muffin cups, filling each about 2/3 full.
7. Bake for 20-25 minutes or until a toothpick inserted into the center comes out clean.
8. Allow the muffins to cool in the tin for 10 minutes before transferring them to a wire rack to cool completely.

Nutrient Facts (per muffin - makes approximately 12):

- Calories: 150
- Carbohydrates: 8g
- Fat: 12g
- Protein: 5g

32. Avocado Lime Sorbet

Prep.Time:	Cook Time:	Serving:	Beverage pairing:
10 min	0 min	6	Herbal Tea

Ingredients:

- 2 ripe avocados
- 1/2 cup fresh lime juice
- Zest of 1 lime
- 1/4 cup sugar-free sweetener (erythritol or stevia)
- 1/2 cup water

Preparation:

1. In a blender or food processor, combine ripe avocados, fresh lime juice, lime zest, sugar-free sweetener, and water.
2. Blend until smooth.
3. Pour the mixture into an ice cream maker and churn according to the manufacturer's instructions.
4. Transfer the sorbet to a shallow dish and freeze for at least 2 hours.
5. Before serving, let the sorbet soften for a few minutes at room temperature and then scoop into bowls.

Nutrient Facts (per serving - 1/2 cup):

- Calories: 120
- Carbohydrates: 7g
- Fat: 10g
- Protein: 2g

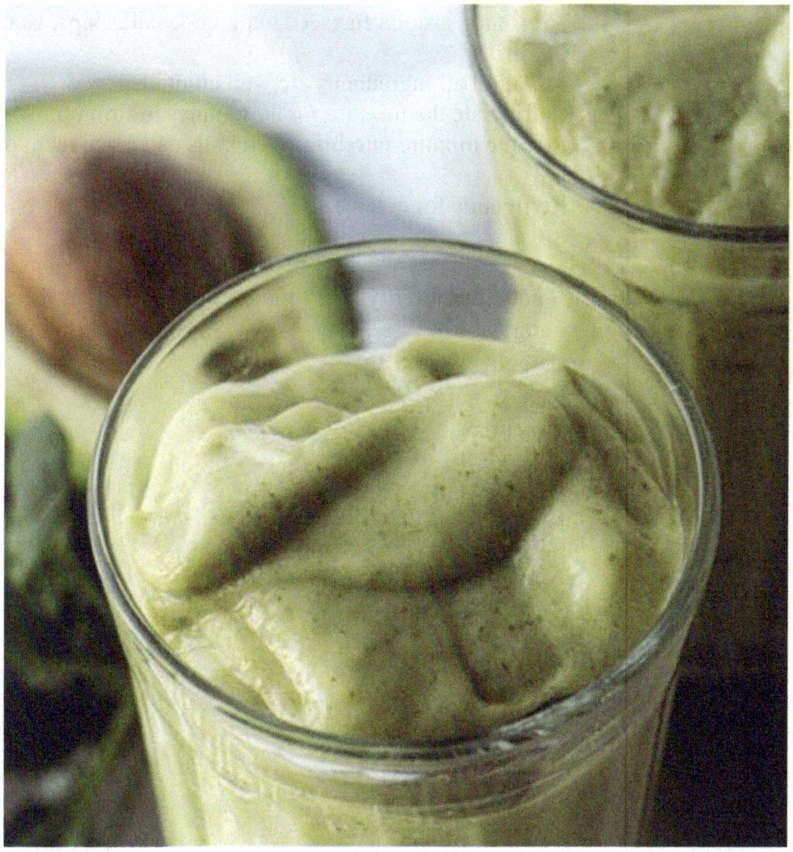

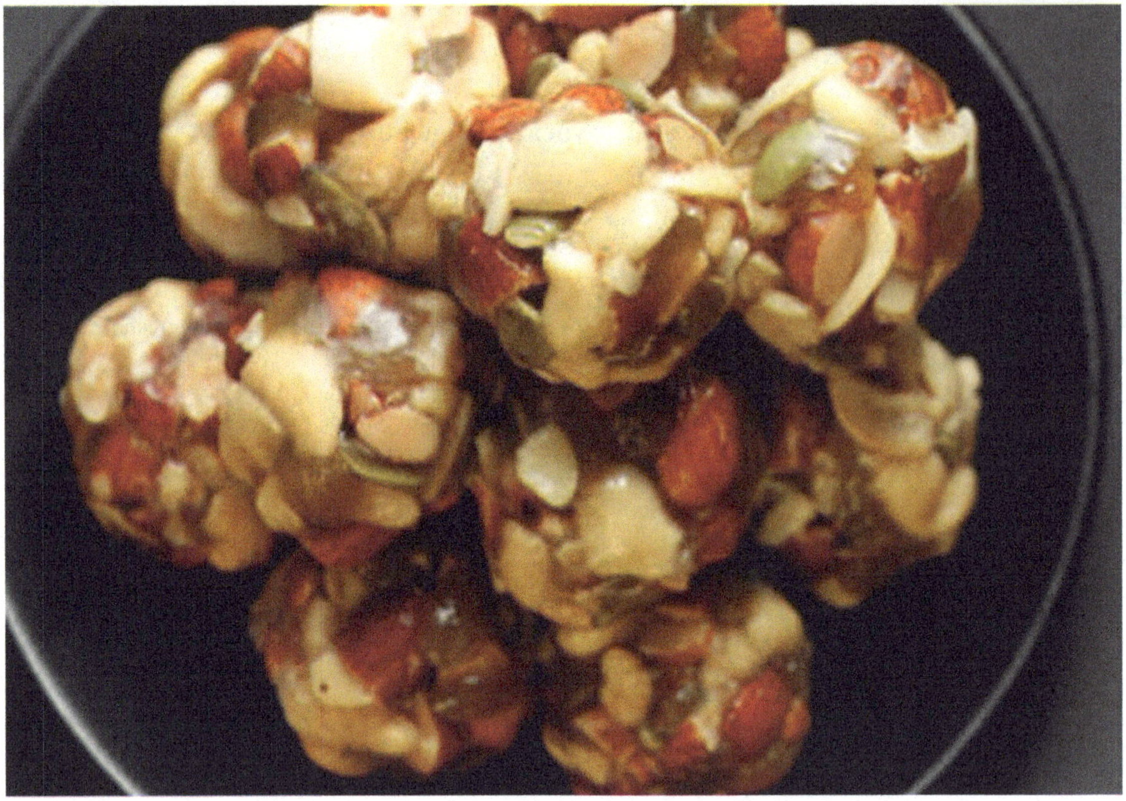

33. No-Bake Almond Butter Energy Bites

Prep.Time: 15 min

Cook Time: 60 min

Serving: 12

Beverage pairing: Almond Milk

Ingredients:

- 1 cup rolled oats
- 1/2 cup almond butter
- 1/4 cup honey or sugar-free sweetener
- 1/2 cup ground flaxseed
- 1/2 cup dark chocolate chips (sugar-free or at least 70% cocoa)
- 1 teaspoon vanilla extract
- A pinch of salt

Preparation:

1. In a bowl, combine rolled oats, almond butter, honey or sugar-free sweetener, ground flaxseed, dark chocolate chips, vanilla extract, and a pinch of salt.
2. Mix until all ingredients are well combined.
3. Refrigerate the mixture for 30 minutes to firm up.
4. Roll the mixture into bite-sized balls and place them on a parchment-lined tray.
5. Refrigerate for at least 1 hour before serving.

Nutrient Facts (per energy bite - makes approximately 12):

- Calories: 120
- Carbohydrates: 12g
- Fat: 7g
- Protein: 3g

34. Coconut Flour Zucchini Brownies

Prep.Time: 15 min

Cook Time: 30 min

Serving: 12

Beverage pairing: Herbal Tea

Ingredients:

- 1 cup shredded zucchini, squeezed to remove excess moisture
- 1/2 cup coconut flour
- 1/2 cup cocoa powder (unsweetened)
- 1/4 teaspoon baking soda
- 1/4 teaspoon salt
- 1/4 cup melted coconut oil
- 1/4 cup sugar-free sweetener (erythritol or stevia)
- 3 large eggs
- 1 teaspoon vanilla extract
- 1/2 cup dark chocolate chips (sugar-free or at least 70% cocoa)

Preparation:

1. Preheat the oven to 350°F (175°C) and line a baking dish with parchment paper.
2. In a bowl, combine shredded zucchini, coconut flour, cocoa powder, baking soda, and salt.
3. In another bowl, whisk together melted coconut oil, sugar-free sweetener, eggs, and vanilla extract.
4. Add the wet ingredients to the dry ingredients and mix until well combined.
5. Fold in dark chocolate chips.
6. Spread the batter evenly in the prepared baking dish.
7. Bake for 25-30 minutes or until a toothpick inserted into the center comes out with moist crumbs (not wet batter).
8. Allow the brownies to cool in the dish before cutting into squares.

Nutrient Facts (per brownie - makes approximately 12):

- Calories: 120
- Carbohydrates: 10g
- Fat: 8g
- Protein: 3g

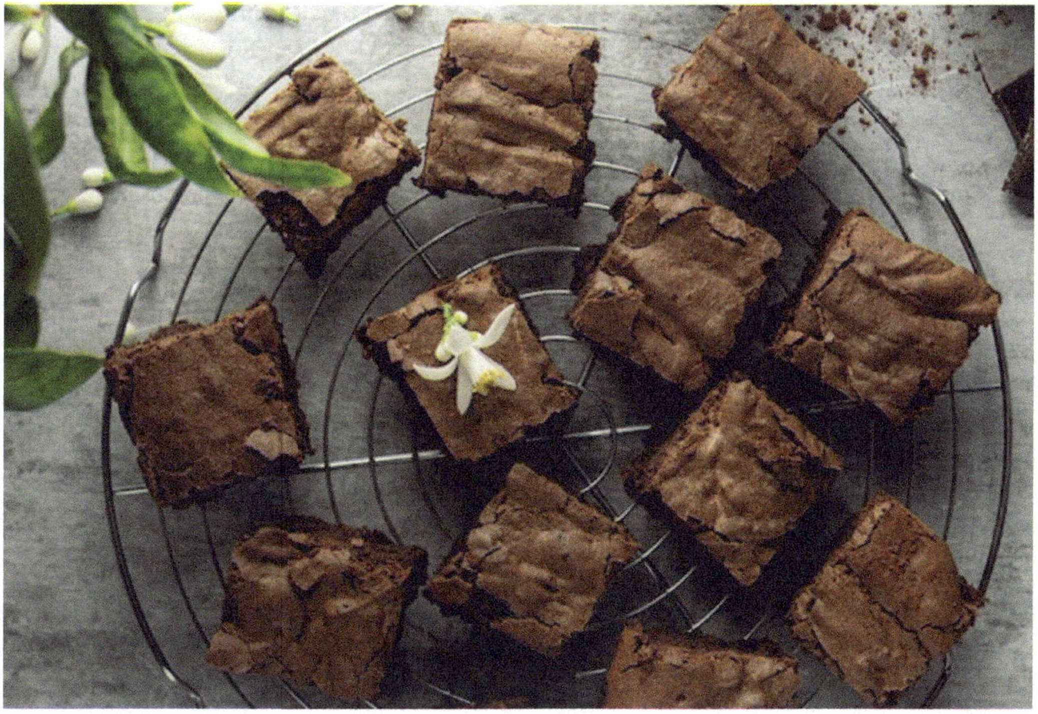

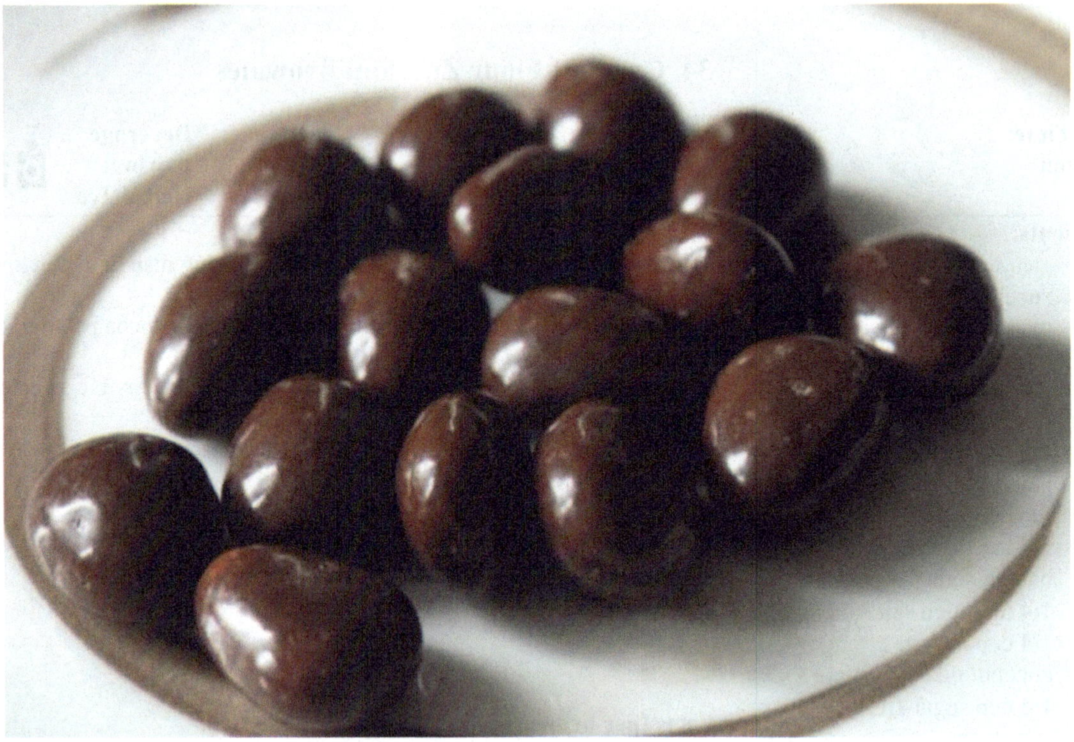

35. Dark Chocolate-Covered Almond Clusters

Prep.Time:	Cook Time:	Serving:	Beverage pairing:
10 min	60 min	12	Black Coffee

Ingredients:

- 1 cup raw almonds
- 1/2 cup dark chocolate chips (sugar-free or at least 70% cocoa)
- 1 tablespoon coconut oil
- 1/4 teaspoon sea salt

Preparation:

1. In a dry skillet over medium heat, toast the almonds until fragrant, about 5-7 minutes. Stir frequently to prevent burning.
2. In a microwave-safe bowl, melt dark chocolate chips and coconut oil in 30-second intervals, stirring between each interval until smooth.
3. Stir the toasted almonds into the melted chocolate, coating them evenly.
4. Spoon clusters of the mixture onto a parchment-lined tray.
5. Sprinkle sea salt over each cluster.
6. Refrigerate for at least 1 hour or until the chocolate is set.

Nutrient Facts (per almond cluster - makes approximately 12):

- Calories: 100
- Carbohydrates: 5g
- Fat: 8g
- Protein: 2g

36. Stevia-Sweetened Berry Smoothie Bowl

Prep.Time: 10 min	**Cook Time:** 0 min	**Serving:** 1	**Beverage pairing:** Herbal Tea

Ingredients:

- 1 cup mixed berries (strawberries, blueberries, raspberries)
- 1/2 frozen banana
- 1/2 cup unsweetened almond milk
- 1 tablespoon chia seeds
- 1/2 teaspoon vanilla extract
- Stevia to taste
- Sliced strawberries
- Blueberries
- Chopped nuts
- Unsweetened shredded coconut

Preparation:

1. In a blender, combine mixed berries, frozen banana, almond milk, chia seeds, vanilla extract, and stevia.
2. Blend until smooth and creamy.
3. Pour the smoothie into a bowl.
4. Top with sliced strawberries, blueberries, chopped nuts, and shredded coconut.

Nutrient Facts (per smoothie bowl):

- Calories: 200
- Carbohydrates: 30g
- Fat: 8g
- Protein: 5g

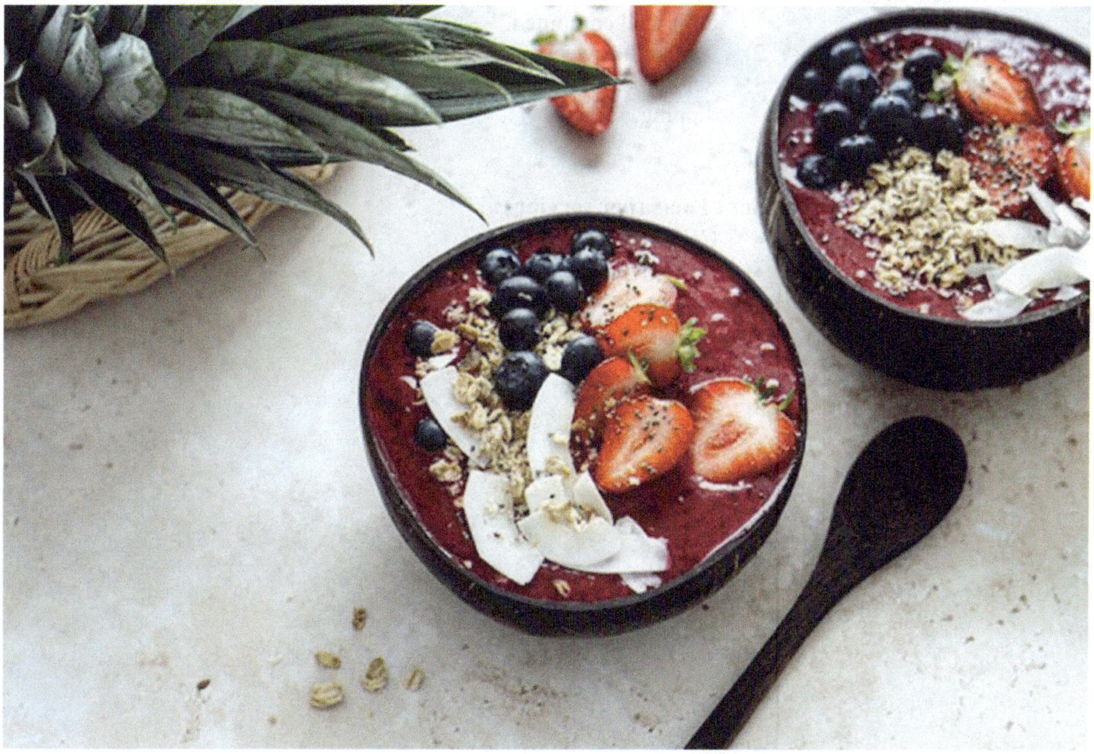

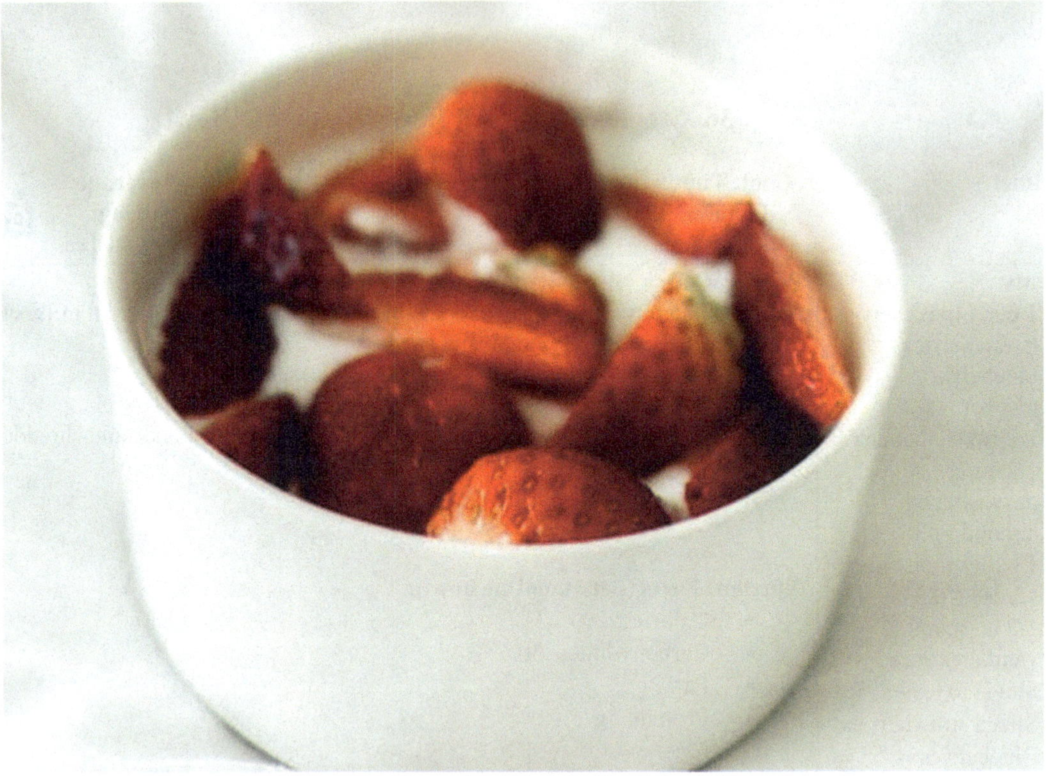

37. Cinnamon Vanilla Greek Yogurt Dip with Sliced Strawberries

Prep.Time: 5 min	**Cook Time:** 0 min	**Serving:** 2	**Beverage pairing:** Herbal Tea

Ingredients:

- 1 cup Greek yogurt (unsweetened)
- 1/2 teaspoon ground cinnamon
- 1/2 teaspoon vanilla extract
- Stevia to taste
- Sliced strawberries for dipping

Preparation:

1. In a bowl, mix Greek yogurt, ground cinnamon, vanilla extract, and stevia until well combined.
2. Adjust the sweetness with more stevia if needed.
3. Serve the cinnamon vanilla Greek yogurt dip with sliced strawberries for dipping.

Nutrient Facts (per serving):

- Calories: 80
- Carbohydrates: 10g
- Fat: 2g
- Protein: 7g

38. Pumpkin Spice Pudding

Prep.Time: 5 min

Cook Time: 0 min

Serving: 2

Beverage pairing: Tea

Ingredients:

- 1/4 cup chia seeds
- 1 cup unsweetened almond milk
- 1/4 cup pumpkin puree
- 1/2 teaspoon pumpkin spice
- Stevia to taste
- Chopped pecans for garnish

Preparation:

1. In a bowl, whisk together chia seeds, almond milk, pumpkin puree, pumpkin spice, and stevia.
2. Refrigerate the mixture for at least 2 hours or overnight, stirring occasionally.
3. Before serving, adjust sweetness with more stevia if needed.
4. Garnish with chopped pecans before serving.

Nutrient Facts (per serving - serves 2):

- Calories: 150
- Carbohydrates: 14g
- Fat: 9g
- Protein: 4g

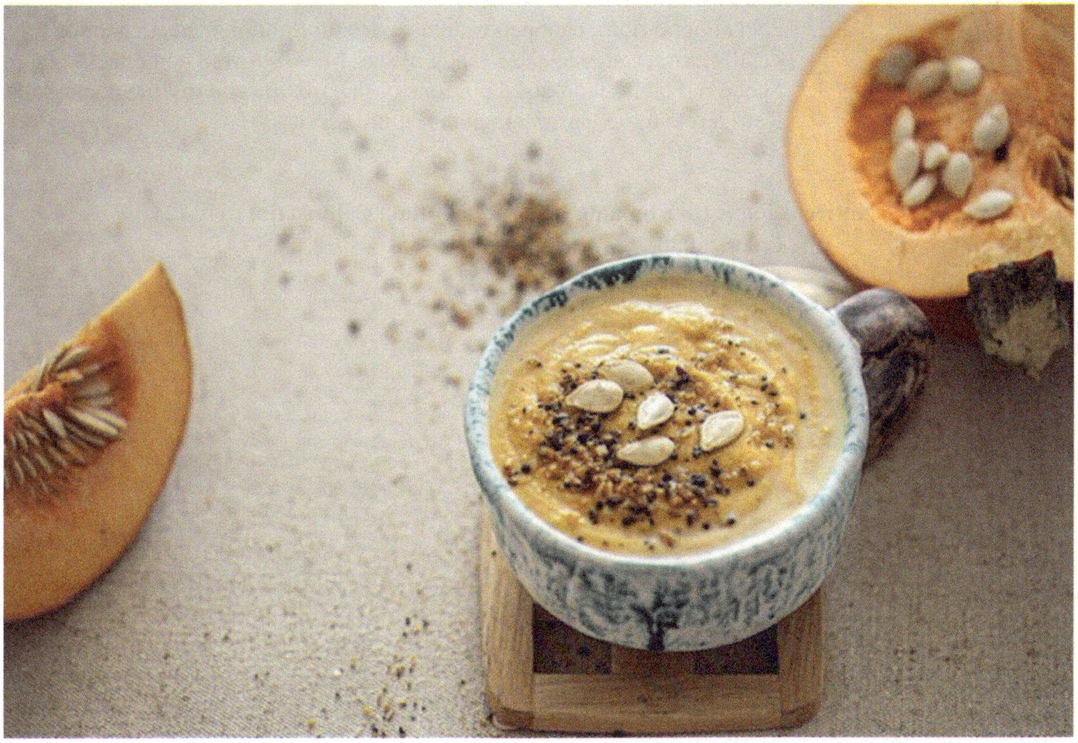

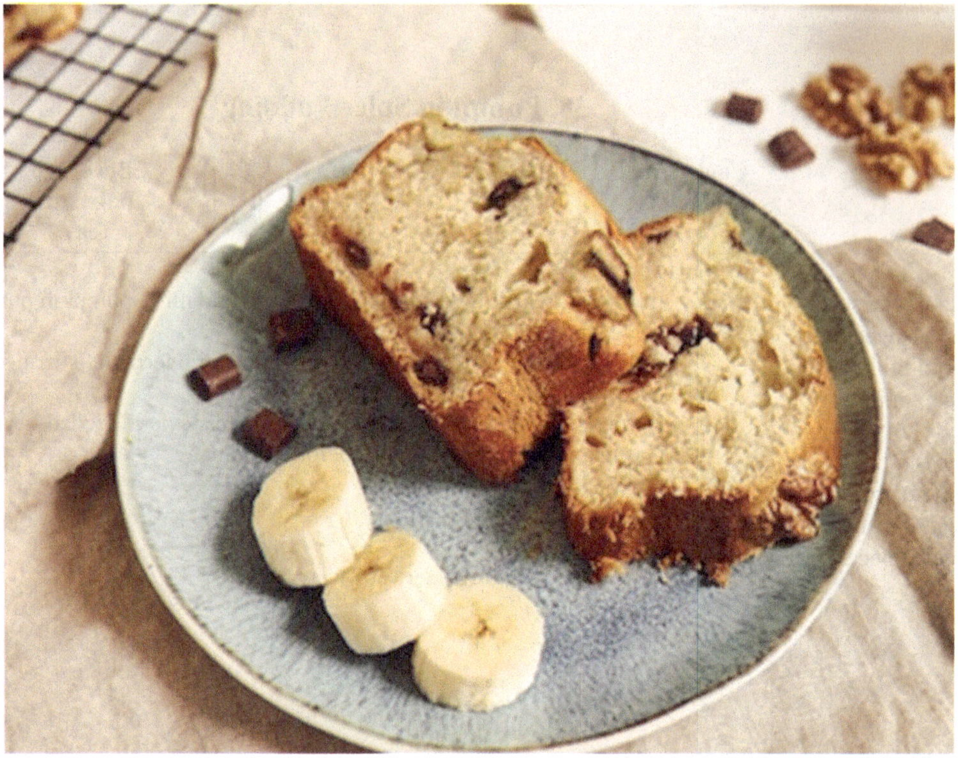

39. Walnut Banana Bread Bites

Prep.Time: 15 min	Cook Time: 30 min	Serving: 12	Beverage pairing: Almond Milk

Ingredients:

- 2 ripe bananas
- 1/4 cup almond flour
- 1/4 cup chopped walnuts
- 1/4 cup coconut flour
- 1/4 cup melted coconut oil
- 1 teaspoon vanilla extract
- Stevia to taste
- A pinch of salt

Preparation:

1. In a bowl, mash ripe bananas.
2. Add almond flour, chopped walnuts, coconut flour, melted coconut oil, vanilla extract, stevia, and a pinch of salt. Mix until well combined.
3. Scoop out tablespoon-sized portions of the mixture and roll them into balls.
4. Refrigerate for at least 30 minutes before serving.

Nutrient Facts (per banana bread bite - makes approximately 12):

- Calories: 80
- Carbohydrates: 8g
- Fat: 5g
- Protein: 1g

40. Blueberry Almond Crumble Bars

Prep.Time: 15 min | **Cook Time:** 30 min | **Serving:** 12 | **Beverage pairing:** Herbal Tea

Ingredients:

- 1 cup almond flour
- 1/4 cup coconut flour
- 1/4 cup melted coconut oil
- Stevia to taste
- 2 cups fresh or frozen blueberries
- 1 tablespoon lemon juice
- 1 tablespoon chia seeds
- 1/2 cup almond flour
- 1/4 cup chopped almonds
- 2 tablespoons melted coconut oil

Preparation:

1. Preheat the oven to 350°F (175°C) and line a baking dish with parchment paper.
2. In a bowl, mix almond flour, coconut flour, melted coconut oil, and stevia to form the crust.
3. Press the crust mixture into the bottom of the prepared baking dish.
4. In another bowl, toss blueberries with lemon juice, chia seeds, and stevia. Spread the blueberry mixture over the crust.
5. In a separate bowl, combine almond flour, chopped almonds, melted coconut oil, and stevia to create the crumble topping.
6. Sprinkle the crumble topping over the blueberry filling.
7. Bake for 25-30 minutes or until the edges are golden brown.
8. Allow the bars to cool in the dish before cutting into squares.

Nutrient Facts (per bar - makes approximately 12):

- Calories: 120
- Carbohydrates: 10g
- Fat: 8g
- Protein: 3g

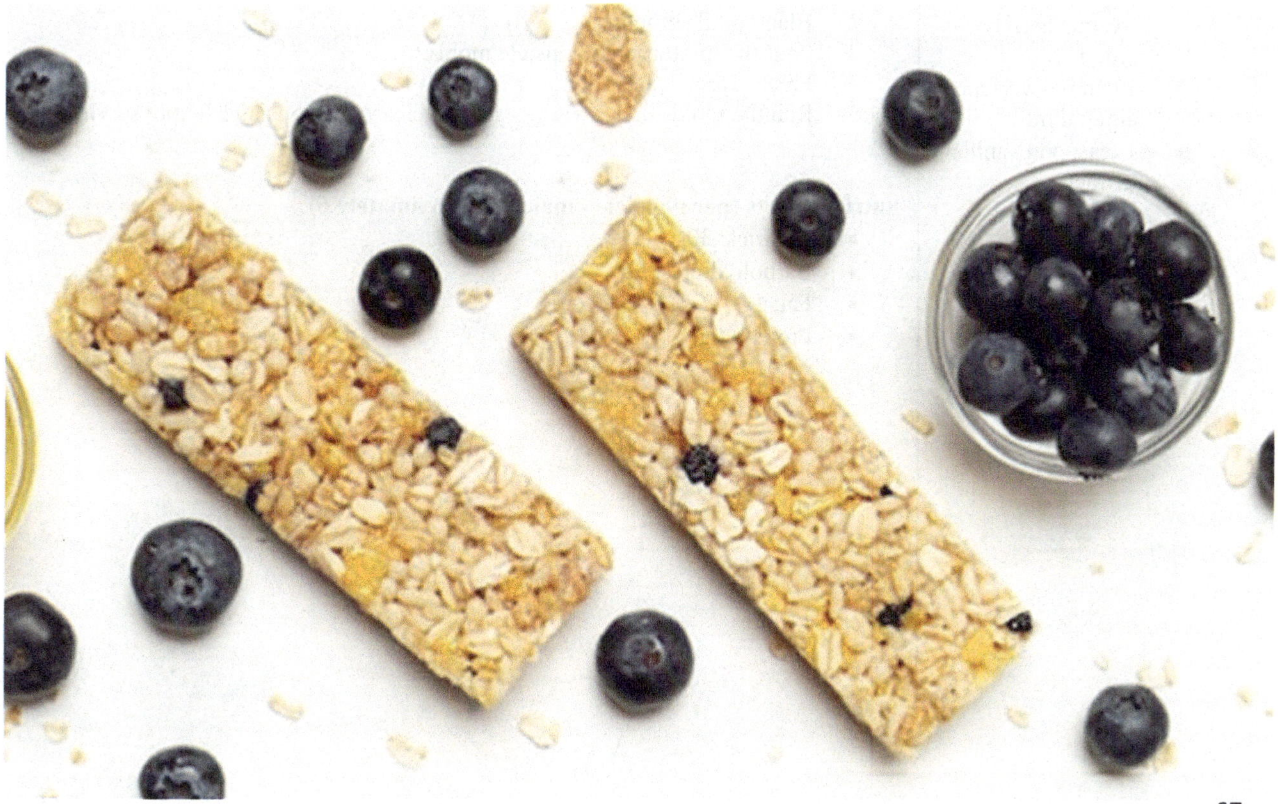

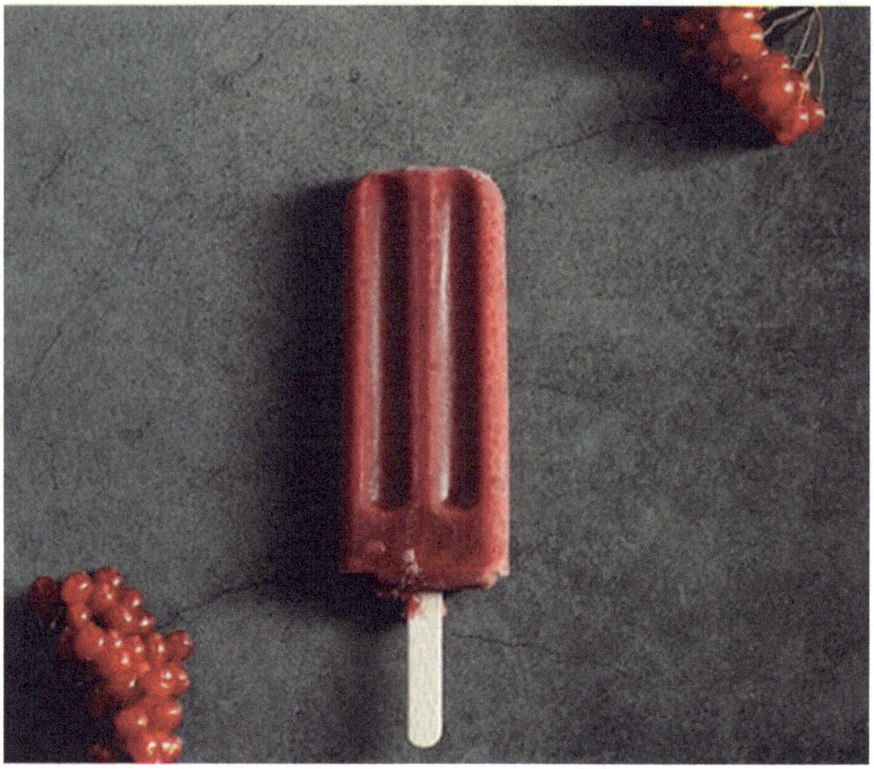

41. Sugar-Free Cherry Vanilla Popsicles

Prep.Time:	Cook Time:	Serving:	Beverage pairing:
10 min	0 min	6	Hibiscus Tea

Ingredients:

- 2 cups fresh or frozen cherries, pitted
- 1 cup unsweetened almond milk
- 1 teaspoon vanilla extract
- Stevia to taste

Preparation:

1. In a blender, combine cherries, almond milk, vanilla extract, and stevia.
2. Blend until smooth.
3. Pour the mixture into popsicle molds.
4. Freeze for at least 4 hours or until fully set.
5. Run the molds under warm water to release the popsicles before serving.

Nutrient Facts (per popsicle - makes approximately 6):

- Calories: 30
- Carbohydrates: 5g
- Fat: 1g
- Protein: 0g

42. Chocolate Chip Cookies

Prep.Time: 15 min	**Cook Time:** 12 min	**Serving:** 12	**Beverage pairing:** hazelnut coffee

Ingredients:

- 2 ripe avocados
- 1/2 cup almond flour
- 1/4 cup coconut flour
- 1/4 cup melted coconut oil
- 1/4 cup sugar-free sweetener (erythritol or stevia)
- 1 teaspoon vanilla extract
- A pinch of salt
- 1/2 cup sugar-free chocolate chips

Preparation:

1. Preheat the oven to 350°F (175°C) and line a baking sheet with parchment paper.
2. In a bowl, mash ripe avocados.
3. Add almond flour, coconut flour, melted coconut oil, sugar-free sweetener, vanilla extract, and a pinch of salt. Mix until well combined.
4. Fold in sugar-free chocolate chips.
5. Drop tablespoon-sized portions of the dough onto the prepared baking sheet.
6. Bake for 10-12 minutes or until the edges are golden brown.
7. Allow the cookies to cool on the baking sheet for 5 minutes before transferring them to a wire rack to cool completely.

Nutrient Facts (per cookie - makes approximately 12):

- Calories: 100
- Carbohydrates: 7g
- Fat: 8g
- Protein: 2g

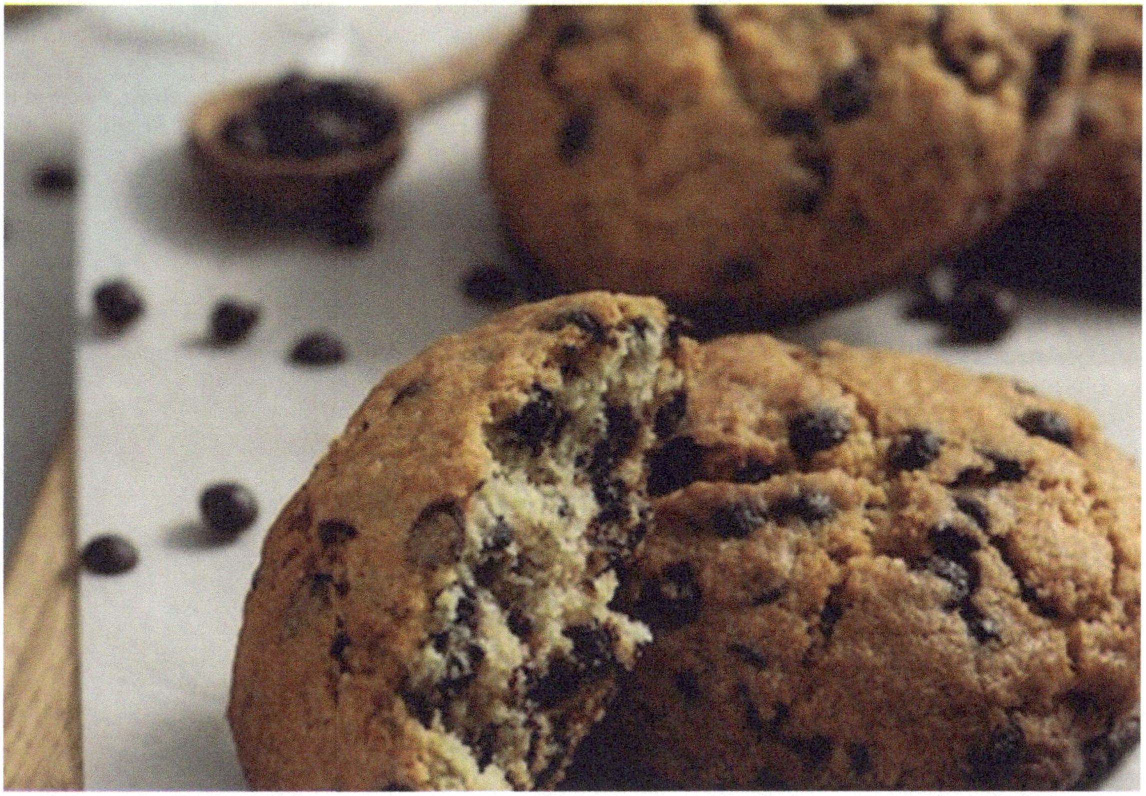

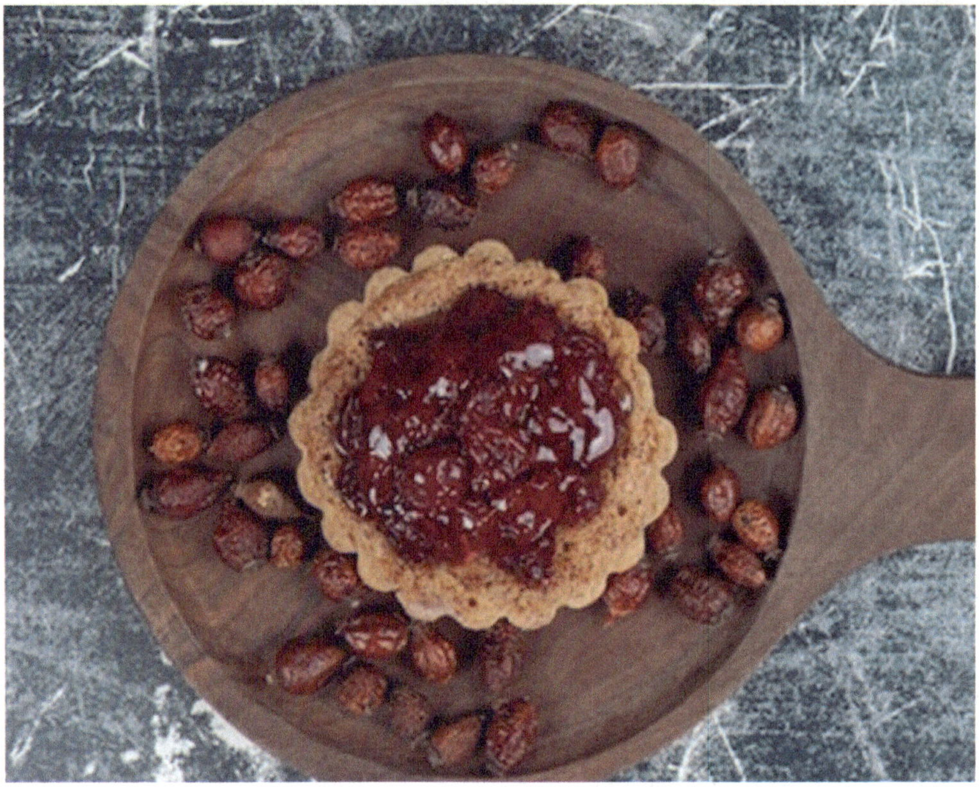

43. No-Sugar Added Raspberry Almond Tart

Prep.Time:	Cook Time:	Serving:	Beverage pairing:
15 min	12 min	8	Iced Tea

Ingredients:

- 1 cup almond flour
- 1/4 cup melted coconut oil
- Stevia to taste
- 1 cup fresh raspberries
- 1/2 cup almond butter
- 1/4 cup coconut milk
- 1 teaspoon vanilla extract

Preparation:

1. Preheat the oven to 350°F (175°C) and line a tart pan with parchment paper.
2. In a bowl, mix almond flour, melted coconut oil, and stevia to form the crust.
3. Press the crust mixture into the bottom of the tart pan.
4. Bake for 10-12 minutes or until the edges are golden brown. Allow it to cool.
5. In a blender, combine raspberries, almond butter, coconut milk, vanilla extract, and stevia. Blend until smooth.
6. Pour the raspberry filling into the cooled crust.
7. Refrigerate for at least 2 hours before serving.

Nutrient Facts (per slice - serves approximately 8):

- Calories: 150
- Carbohydrates: 8g
- Fat: 12g
- Protein: 4g

44. Cocoa-Dusted Pistachios

Prep.Time:	Cook Time:	Serving:	Beverage pairing:
10 min	0 min	8	Black coffee

Ingredients:

- 1 cup raw pistachios
- 2 tablespoons unsweetened cocoa powder
- Stevia to taste

Preparation:

1. In a dry skillet over medium heat, toast the pistachios until they become fragrant, about 5-7 minutes. Stir frequently to prevent burning.
2. In a bowl, combine toasted pistachios, unsweetened cocoa powder, and stevia. Toss until the pistachios are coated.
3. Allow the cocoa-dusted pistachios to cool before serving.

Nutrient Facts (per serving - makes approximately 8):

- Calories: 100
- Carbohydrates: 5g
- Fat: 8g
- Protein: 4g

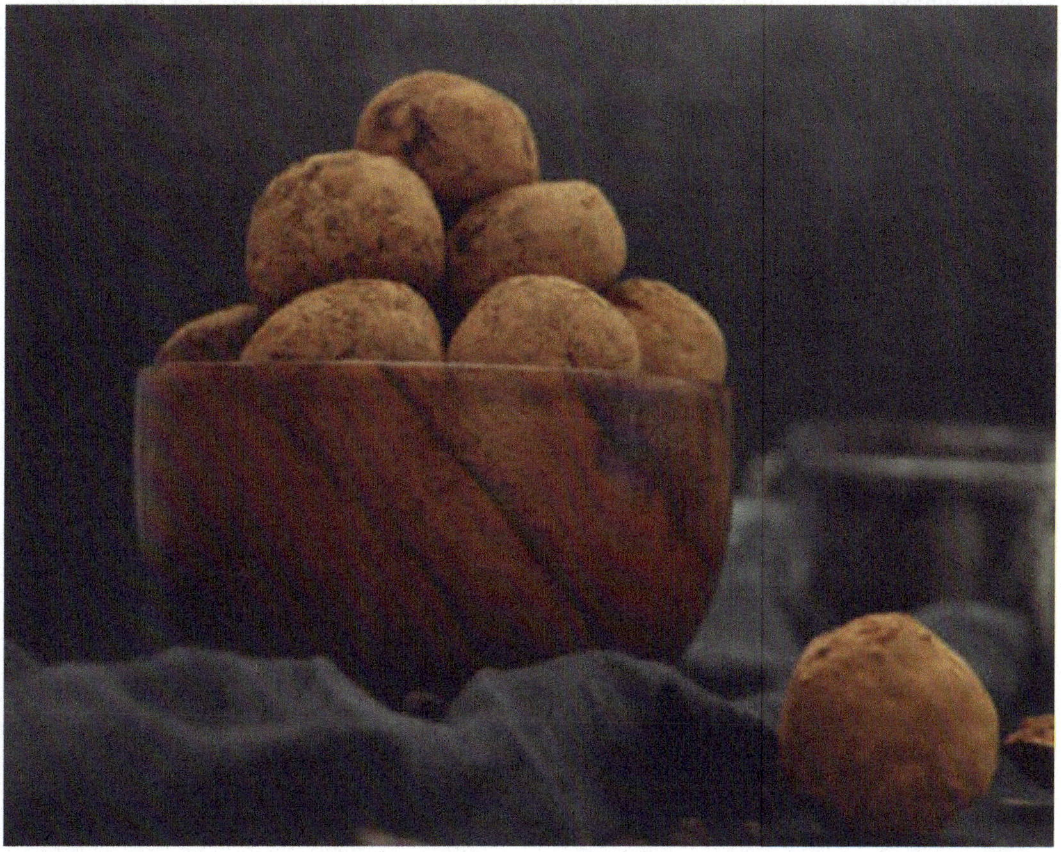

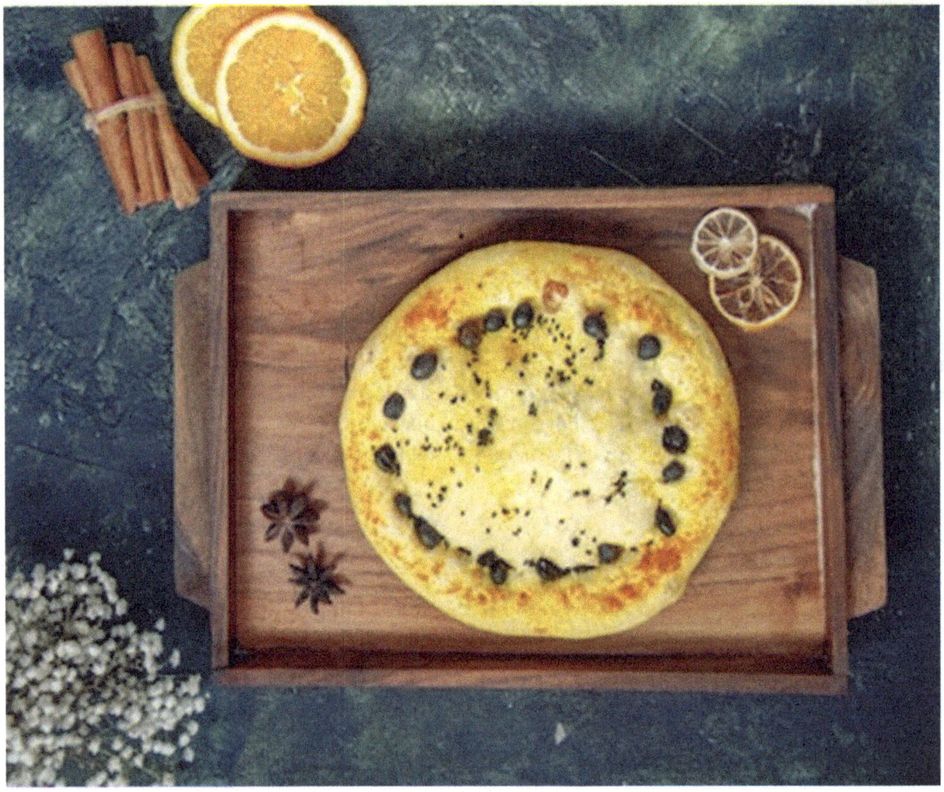

45. Almond Flour Lemon Poppy Seed Cake

Prep.Time: 15 min | **Cook Time:** 30 min | **Serving:** 10 | **Beverage pairing:** Herbal Tea

Ingredients:

- 2 cups almond flour
- 1/4 cup coconut flour
- 1/2 cup melted coconut oil
- 1/2 cup sugar-free sweetener (erythritol or stevia)
- 4 large eggs
- 1/4 cup lemon juice
- Zest of 1 lemon
- 1 teaspoon baking powder
- 1 tablespoon poppy seeds
- 1/4 cup powdered sugar-free sweetener (erythritol or stevia)
- 1 tablespoon lemon juice

Preparation:

1. Preheat the oven to 350°F (175°C) and grease a cake pan.
2. In a bowl, mix almond flour, coconut flour, melted coconut oil, sugar-free sweetener, eggs, lemon juice, lemon zest, baking powder, and poppy seeds until well combined.
3. Pour the batter into the prepared cake pan.
4. Bake for 25-30 minutes or until a toothpick inserted into the center comes out clean.
5. Allow the cake to cool completely.
6. In a small bowl, whisk together powdered sugar-free sweetener and lemon juice to make the glaze.
7. Drizzle the glaze over the cooled cake before serving.

Nutrient Facts (per slice - serves approximately 10):

- Calories: 200
- Carbohydrates: 8g
- Fat: 16g
- Protein: 7g

46. Chocolate Avocado Mousse Parfait

Prep.Time: 10 min

Cook Time: 0 min

Serving: 2

Beverage pairing: Mint Tea

Ingredients:

- 2 ripe avocados
- 1/4 cup cocoa powder (unsweetened)
- 1/4 cup sugar-free sweetener (erythritol or stevia)
- 1 teaspoon vanilla extract
- A pinch of salt
- 1/4 cup unsweetened almond milk
- Sugar-free whipped cream
- Sugar-free chocolate shavings

Preparation:

1. In a blender or food processor, combine ripe avocados, cocoa powder, sugar-free sweetener, vanilla extract, a pinch of salt, and unsweetened almond milk.
2. Blend until smooth and creamy.
3. Spoon the chocolate avocado mousse into serving glasses.
4. Alternate layers of mousse with sugar-free whipped cream in parfait glasses.
5. Top with sugar-free chocolate shavings before serving.

Nutrient Facts (per parfait - serves approximately 2):

- Calories: 200
- Carbohydrates: 15g
- Fat: 15g
- Protein: 4g

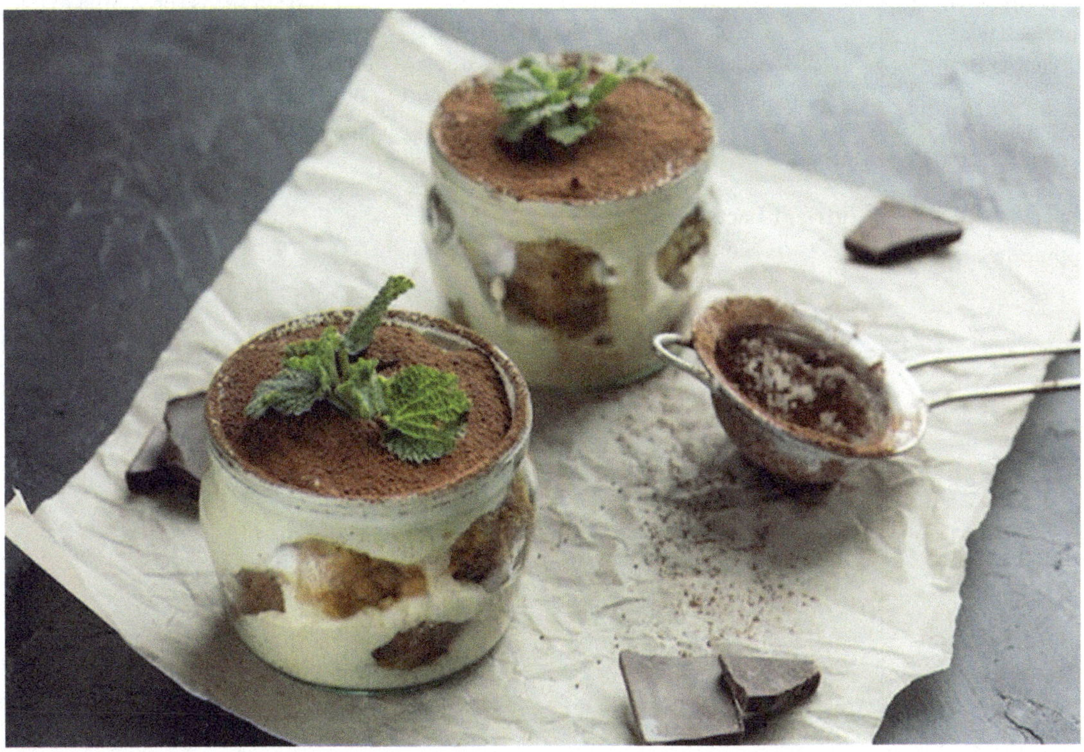

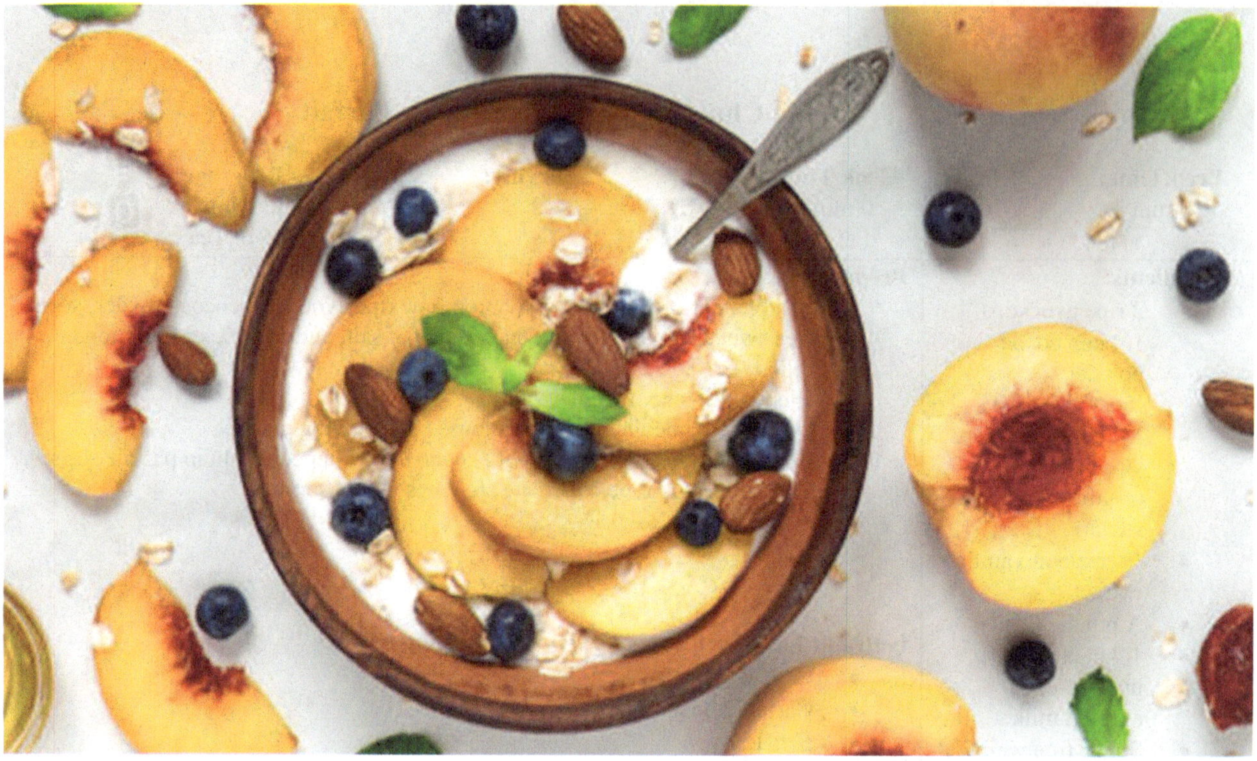

47. Greek Yogurt with Sliced Peaches

Prep.Time:	Cook Time:	Serving:	Beverage pairing:
5 min	0 min	2	Green Tea

Ingredients:

- 1 cup Greek yogurt (unsweetened)
- 1/2 vanilla bean, seeds scraped (or 1 teaspoon vanilla extract)
- Stevia to taste
- Sliced peaches for topping

Preparation:

1. In a bowl, mix Greek yogurt, scraped vanilla bean seeds (or vanilla extract), and stevia until well combined.
2. Adjust sweetness with more stevia if needed.
3. Serve the vanilla bean Greek yogurt in bowls and top with sliced peaches.

Nutrient Facts (per serving):

- Calories: 100
- Carbohydrates: 10g
- Fat: 2g
- Protein: 15g

48. No-Bake Coconut Almond Energy Balls

Prep.Time:	Cook Time:	Serving:	Beverage pairing:
15 min	0 min	12	Herbal Tea

Ingredients:

- 1 cup rolled oats
- 1/2 cup almond butter
- 1/4 cup honey or sugar-free sweetener
- 1/4 cup shredded coconut (unsweetened)
- 1/4 cup chopped almonds
- 1 teaspoon vanilla extract
- A pinch of salt

Preparation:

1. In a bowl, combine rolled oats, almond butter, honey or sugar-free sweetener, shredded coconut, chopped almonds, vanilla extract, and a pinch of salt.
2. Mix until all ingredients are well combined.
3. Refrigerate the mixture for 30 minutes to firm up.
4. Roll the mixture into bite-sized balls and place them on a parchment-lined tray.
5. Refrigerate for at least 1 hour before serving.

Nutrient Facts (per energy ball - makes approximately 12):

- Calories: 100
- Carbohydrates: 10g
- Fat: 6g
- Protein: 3g

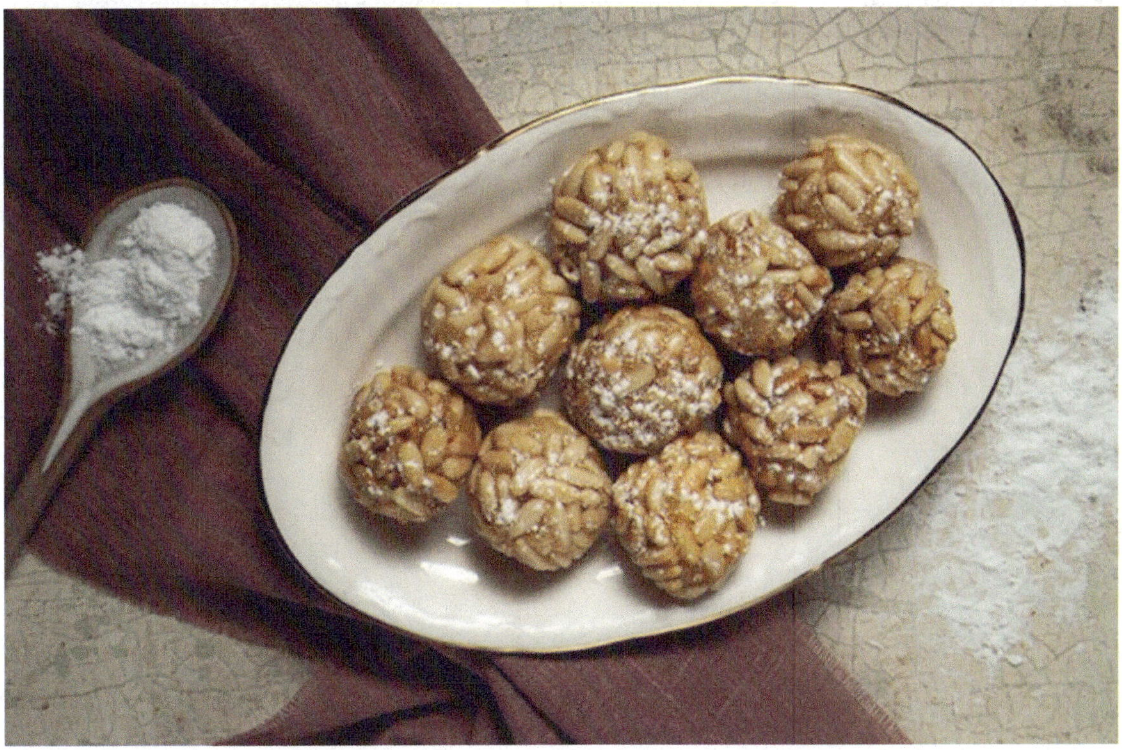

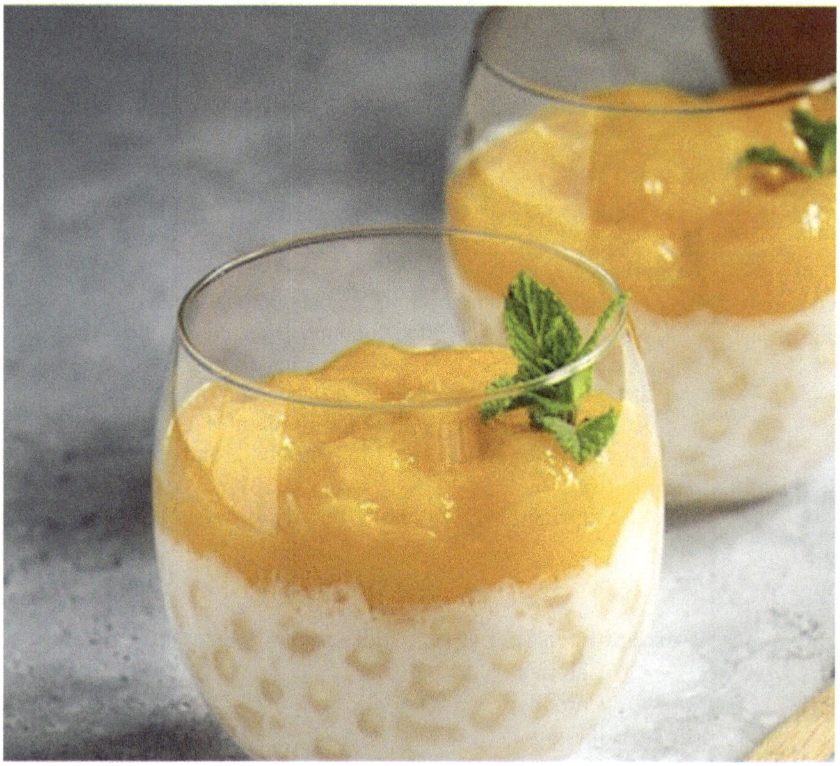

49. Sugar-Free Mango Coconut Chia Pudding

Prep.Time:	Cook Time:	Serving:	Beverage pairing:
5 min	0 min	2	Iced Tea

Ingredients:

- 1/4 cup chia seeds
- 1 cup unsweetened coconut milk
- 1/2 cup fresh mango, diced
- Stevia to taste
- Shredded coconut for garnish

Preparation:

1. In a bowl, whisk together chia seeds, coconut milk, diced mango, and stevia.
2. Refrigerate the mixture for at least 2 hours or overnight, stirring occasionally.
3. Before serving, adjust sweetness with more stevia if needed.
4. Garnish with shredded coconut before serving.

Nutrient Facts (per serving - serves 2):

- Calories: 150
- Carbohydrates: 12g
- Fat: 10g
- Protein: 4g

50. Strawberry Rhubarb Crisp

Prep.Time:	Cook Time:	Serving:	Beverage pairing:
15 min	30 min	6	Iced Tea

Ingredients:

- 2 cups fresh strawberries, sliced
- 1 cup rhubarb, diced
- Stevia to taste
- 1 tablespoon lemon juice
- 1 tablespoon arrowroot powder (or cornstarch)
- 1 cup almond flour
- 1/4 cup melted coconut oil
- Stevia to taste
- 1/2 cup chopped pecans

Preparation:

1. Preheat the oven to 350°F (175°C) and grease a baking dish.
2. In a bowl, combine sliced strawberries, diced rhubarb, stevia, lemon juice, and arrowroot powder. Toss until well coated.
3. In another bowl, mix almond flour, melted coconut oil, stevia, and chopped pecans to create the crumble topping.
4. Spread the strawberry-rhubarb mixture evenly in the prepared baking dish.
5. Sprinkle the crumble topping over the fruit.
6. Bake for 30-35 minutes or until the topping is golden brown and the filling is bubbly.
7. Allow the crisp to cool for a few minutes before serving.

Nutrient Facts (per serving - serves approximately 6):

- Calories: 200
- Carbohydrates: 15g
- Fat: 16g
- Protein: 4g

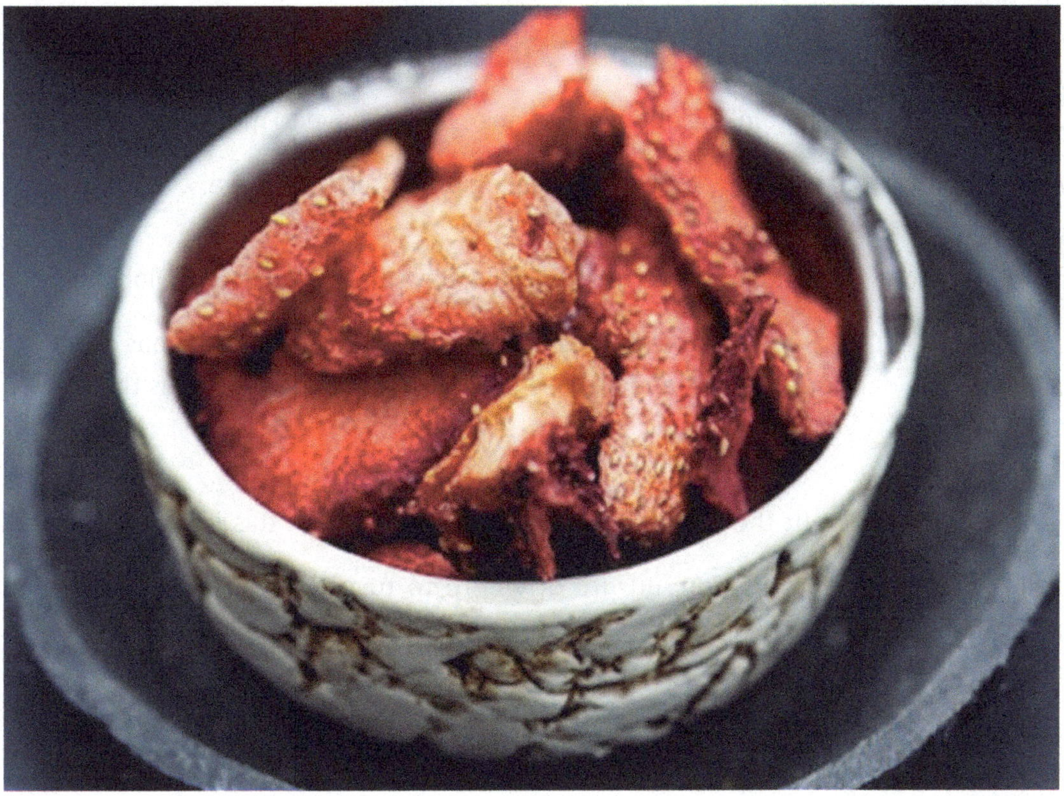

Your Kindness is Key

Share Your Experience, Share Your Strength

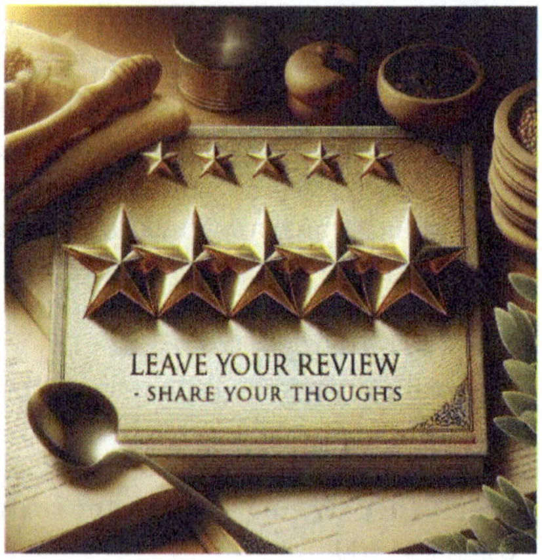

"Helping one person might not change the whole world, but it could change the world for one person." - Anonymous

---

Do you remember what it was like when you first heard the words "Type 2 Diabetes?" Perhaps it felt like a mountain you weren't sure you could climb.

Maybe it was daunting, thinking about the changes you'd have to make in your life, especially with your diet. It's a journey many embark on feeling uncertain and alone.

But you've found a companion on this journey, haven't you? Type 2 Diabetes Cookbook Beginner's Quick & Easy Recipes for Delicious Diabetes Diets by Lily Anders has been with you, offering guidance, delicious recipes, and a sense of control over your diabetes that perhaps you didn't feel before.

Imagine if you could light the path for someone just starting on this journey. Someone who feels lost in the sea of information, unsure of where to turn for reliable, practical advice on managing their diabetes through diet. Your experience, shared through a review, could be the beacon they need.

This isn't just about leaving a review; it's about extending a hand, offering support, and sharing the strength that comes from knowledge and community. Your words could help another person find their footing, making their journey a bit easier and less lonely.

So, here's my humble request on behalf of a fellow journeyer you've yet to meet:

Please take a moment to share your experience with the book. Your insights could be the very thing another person needs to hear to take that first, brave step toward a healthier, happier life with diabetes. Your review, a simple act of kindness, asks for nothing in return yet offers immeasurable value.

To leave your review, just follow this link:

https://www.amazon.com/review/create-review/?ie=UTF8&channel=glance-detail&asin=1963939328

If the thought of helping another soul on their diabetes journey warms your heart, then you're exactly who I hoped to reach with this book. Welcome to a community where kindness, support, and shared victories pave the way to a better life.

I'm beyond grateful for your help in spreading the word and even more excited to continue providing you with the knowledge and recipes to make managing diabetes not just manageable, but enjoyable.

Click the QR Code Here!

Thank you from the deepest places in my heart. Your generosity makes all the difference.

Lily Anders

P.S. - Sharing is caring, they say. If you believe this book has brought value to your life and could do the same for someone else, consider sharing it with them. It's another beautiful way to change a life, one meal at a time.

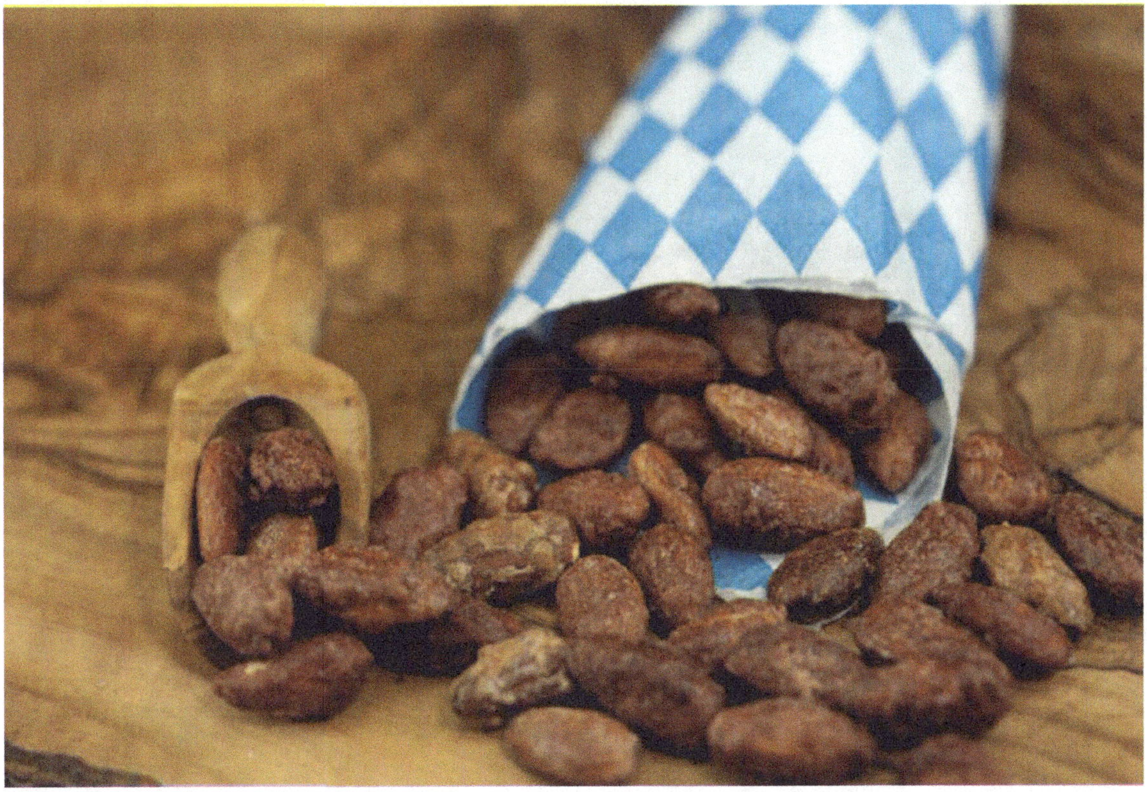

51. Cinnamon Roasted Almond Slices

Prep.Time: 5 min

Cook Time: 12 min

Serving: 4

Beverage pairing: Tea

Ingredients:

- 1 cup almond slices
- 1 tablespoon melted coconut oil
- 1 teaspoon ground cinnamon
- Stevia to taste

Preparation:

1. Preheat the oven to 325°F (163°C) and line a baking sheet with parchment paper.
2. In a bowl, toss almond slices with melted coconut oil, ground cinnamon, and stevia.
3. Spread the almonds in a single layer on the prepared baking sheet.
4. Roast for 10-12 minutes or until golden brown, stirring halfway through.
5. Allow the cinnamon roasted almond slices to cool completely before serving.

Nutrient Facts (per serving - makes approximately 1 cup):

- Calories: 120
- Carbohydrates: 4g
- Fat: 10g
- Protein: 4g

52. Peanut Butter Banana Ice Cream

Prep.Time: 5 min

Cook Time: 0 min

Serving: 2

Beverage pairing: Almond Milk

Ingredients:

- 2 ripe bananas, sliced and frozen
- 2 tablespoons peanut butter (unsweetened)
- Stevia to taste
- Chopped peanuts for topping (optional)

Preparation:

1. In a blender or food processor, combine frozen banana slices, peanut butter, and stevia.
2. Blend until smooth and creamy.
3. Adjust sweetness with more stevia if needed.
4. Transfer the ice cream to a bowl and top with chopped peanuts if desired.

Nutrient Facts (per serving):

- Calories: 150
- Carbohydrates: 20g
- Fat: 7g
- Protein: 3g

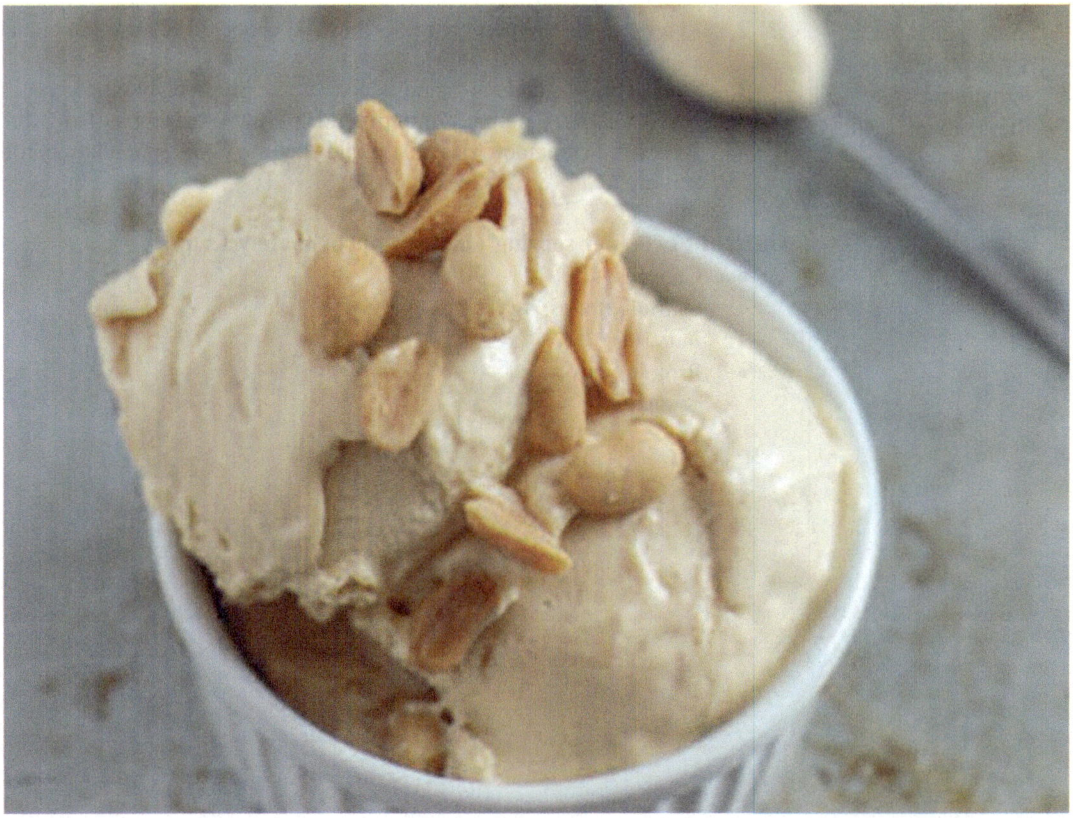

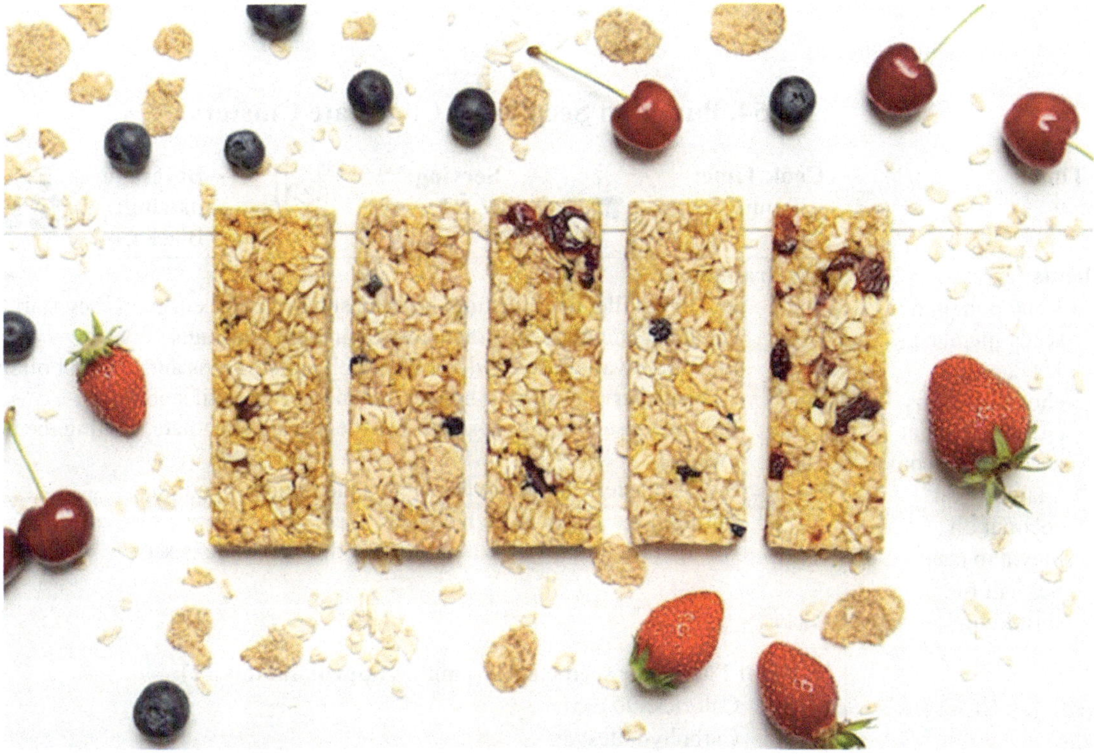

53. Cherry Almond Protein Bars

Prep.Time:	Cook Time:	Serving:	Beverage pairing:
15 min	0 min	8	Herbal Tea

Ingredients:

- 1 cup almonds
- 1 cup dried cherries (unsweetened)
- 1/4 cup protein powder (vanilla or unflavored)
- 2 tablespoons almond butter (unsweetened)
- Stevia to taste
- Water (as needed)

Preparation:

1. In a food processor, blend almonds until finely ground.
2. Add dried cherries, protein powder, almond butter, and stevia. Blend until the mixture starts to come together.
3. If the mixture is too dry, add water a tablespoon at a time until it sticks together.
4. Press the mixture into a lined pan and refrigerate for at least 1 hour.
5. Cut into bars before serving.

Nutrient Facts (per bar - makes approximately 8):

- Calories: 150
- Carbohydrates: 15g
- Fat: 9g
- Protein: 5g

54. Pumpkin Seed Dark Chocolate Clusters

Prep.Time: 10 min

Cook Time: 0 min

Serving: 12

Beverage pairing: Black Coffee

Ingredients:

- 1 cup pumpkin seeds (pepitas)
- 1/2 cup dark chocolate chips (sugar-free or at least 70% cocoa)
- 1 tablespoon coconut oil
- Stevia to taste
- Sea salt for sprinkling

Preparation:

1. In a dry skillet over medium heat, toast pumpkin seeds until they start to pop, about 5-7 minutes. Stir frequently to prevent burning.
2. In a microwave-safe bowl, melt dark chocolate chips and coconut oil in 30-second intervals, stirring between each interval until smooth.
3. Stir the toasted pumpkin seeds into the melted chocolate, coating them evenly.
4. Spoon clusters of the mixture onto a parchment-lined tray.
5. Sprinkle sea salt over each cluster.
6. Refrigerate for at least 1 hour or until the chocolate is set.

Nutrient Facts (per seed cluster - makes approximately 12):

- Calories: 90
- Carbohydrates: 5g
- Fat: 7g
- Protein: 2g

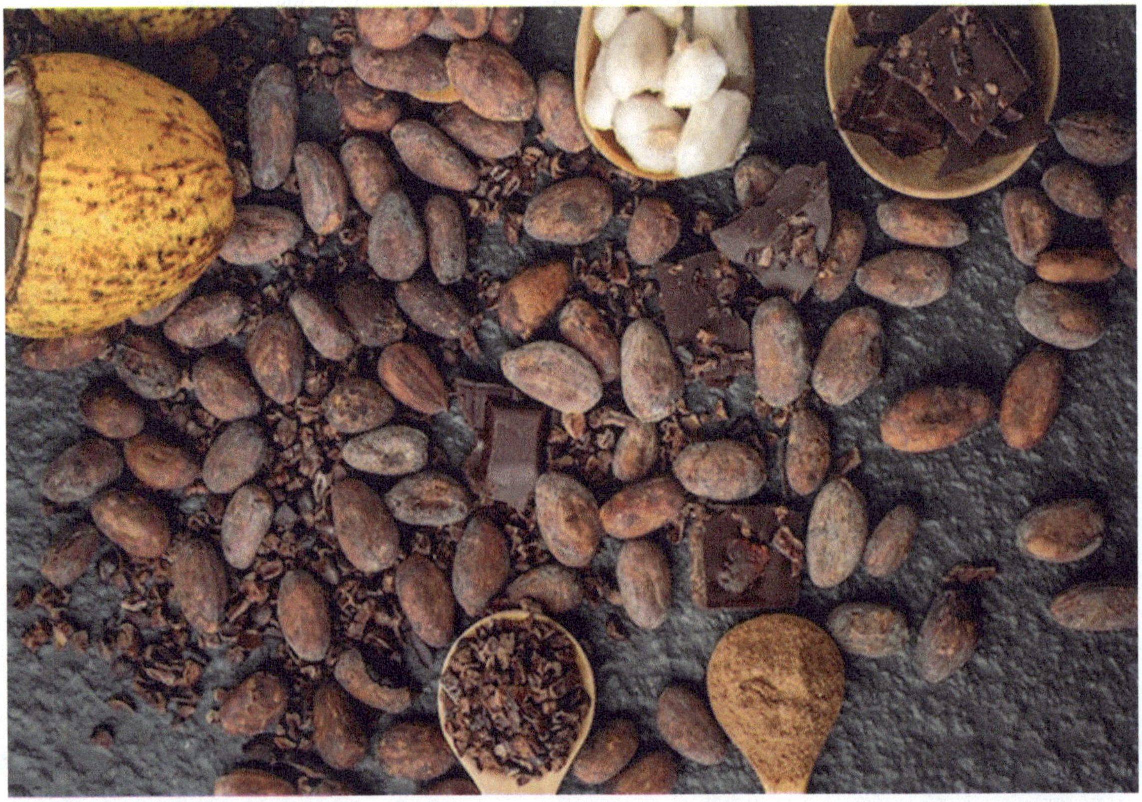

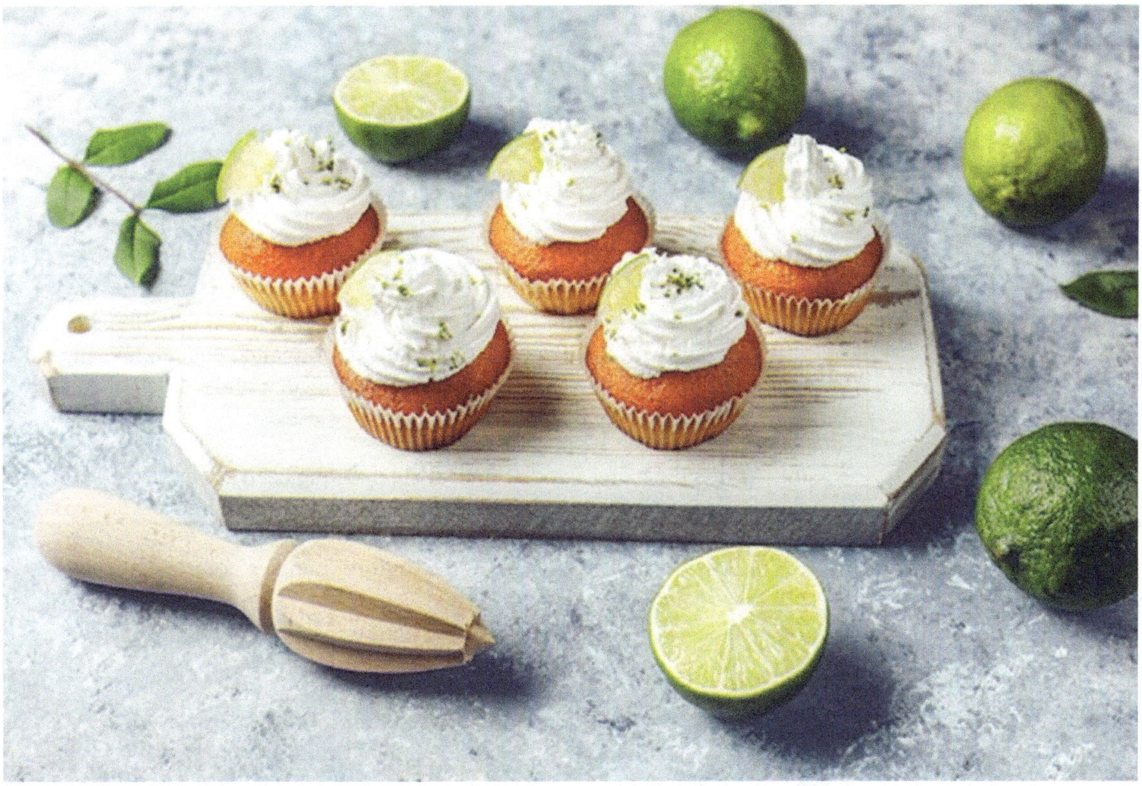

55. No-Sugar Added Lemon Ricotta Cheesecake Cups

Prep.Time: 10 min	Cook Time: 0 min	Serving: 4	Beverage pairing: Chamomile Tea

Ingredients:

- 1 cup ricotta cheese (full-fat)
- 1/4 cup almond flour
- 2 tablespoons lemon juice
- Zest of 1 lemon
- Stevia to taste
- Fresh berries for topping (optional)

Preparation:

1. In a bowl, mix ricotta cheese, almond flour, lemon juice, lemon zest, and stevia until well combined.
2. Adjust sweetness with more stevia if needed.
3. Spoon the lemon ricotta mixture into serving cups.
4. Refrigerate for at least 2 hours before serving.
5. Top with fresh berries before serving if desired.

Nutrient Facts (per cup - makes approximately 4):

- Calories: 150
- Carbohydrates: 5g
- Fat: 12g
- Protein: 8g

56. Almond Flour Blackberry Muffins

Prep.Time:	Cook Time:	Serving:	Beverage pairing:
10 min	20 min	12	Green Tea

Ingredients:

- 2 cups almond flour
- 1/4 cup coconut flour
- 1/4 cup melted coconut oil
- 1/4 cup sugar-free sweetener (erythritol or stevia)
- 3 large eggs
- 1 teaspoon vanilla extract
- 1/2 teaspoon baking powder
- A pinch of salt
- 1 cup fresh blackberries

Preparation:

1. Preheat the oven to 350°F (175°C) and line a muffin tin with paper liners.
2. In a bowl, mix almond flour, coconut flour, melted coconut oil, sugar-free sweetener, eggs, vanilla extract, baking powder, and a pinch of salt until well combined.
3. Gently fold in fresh blackberries.
4. Spoon the batter into the muffin cups, filling each about 2/3 full.
5. Bake for 20-25 minutes or until a toothpick inserted into the center comes out clean.
6. Allow the muffins to cool in the tin for 5 minutes before transferring them to a wire rack to cool completely.

Nutrient Facts (per muffin - makes approximately 12):

- Calories: 150
- Carbohydrates: 8g
- Fat: 12g
- Protein: 5g

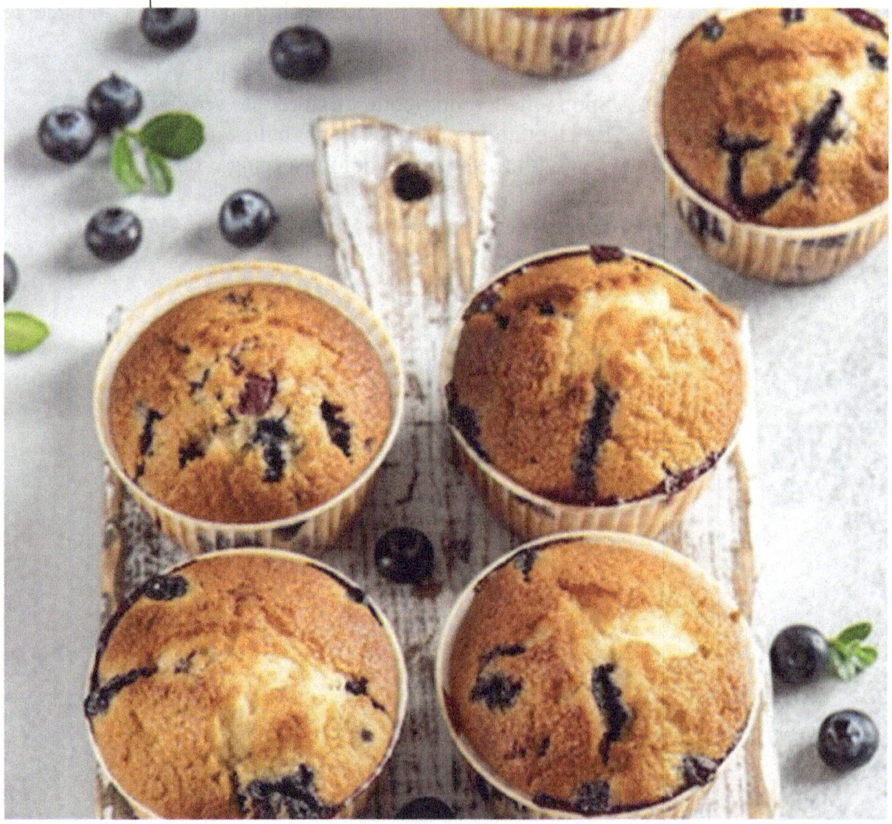

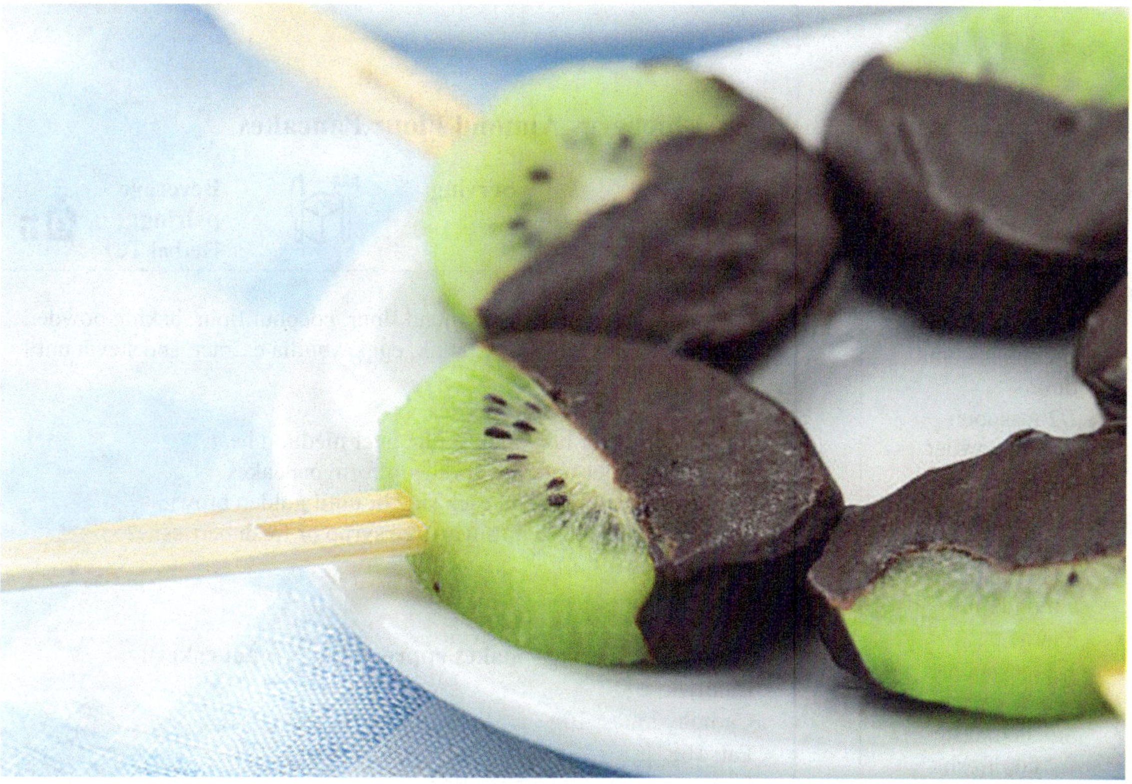

57. Chocolate Covered Kiwi Slices

Prep.Time: 15 min	**Cook Time:** 30 min	**Serving:** 3	**Beverage pairing:** Green Tea

Ingredients:

- 3 kiwis, peeled and sliced
- 1/2 cup dark chocolate chips (sugar-free or at least 70% cocoa)
- 1 tablespoon coconut oil
- Stevia to taste
- Chopped nuts for garnish (optional)

Preparation:

1. In a microwave-safe bowl, melt dark chocolate chips and coconut oil in 30-second intervals, stirring between each interval until smooth.
2. Dip kiwi slices into the melted chocolate, coating them halfway.
3. Place the chocolate-covered kiwi slices on a parchment-lined tray.
4. Sprinkle chopped nuts over the chocolate if desired.
5. Refrigerate for at least 30 minutes or until the chocolate is set.

Nutrient Facts (per serving - serves approximately 3):

- Calories: 120
- Carbohydrates: 12g
- Fat: 8g
- Protein: 2g

58. Blueberry Almond Flour Pancakes

Prep.Time:	Cook Time:	Serving:	Beverage pairing:
10 min	12 min	3	Herbal Tea

Ingredients:

- 1 cup almond flour
- 1/4 cup coconut flour
- 1/2 teaspoon baking powder
- 1/4 cup melted coconut oil
- 1/4 cup unsweetened almond milk
- 3 large eggs
- 1/2 teaspoon vanilla extract
- Stevia to taste
- 1/2 cup fresh blueberries

Preparation:

1. In a bowl, whisk together almond flour, coconut flour, baking powder, melted coconut oil, almond milk, eggs, vanilla extract, and stevia until smooth.
2. Gently fold in fresh blueberries.
3. Heat a griddle or non-stick skillet over medium heat.
4. Spoon the batter onto the griddle to form pancakes.
5. Cook for 2-3 minutes on each side or until golden brown.
6. Serve the pancakes with sugar-free syrup or fresh berries.

Nutrient Facts (per serving - makes approximately 6 pancakes):

- Calories: 200
- Carbohydrates: 10g
- Fat: 16g
- Protein: 7g

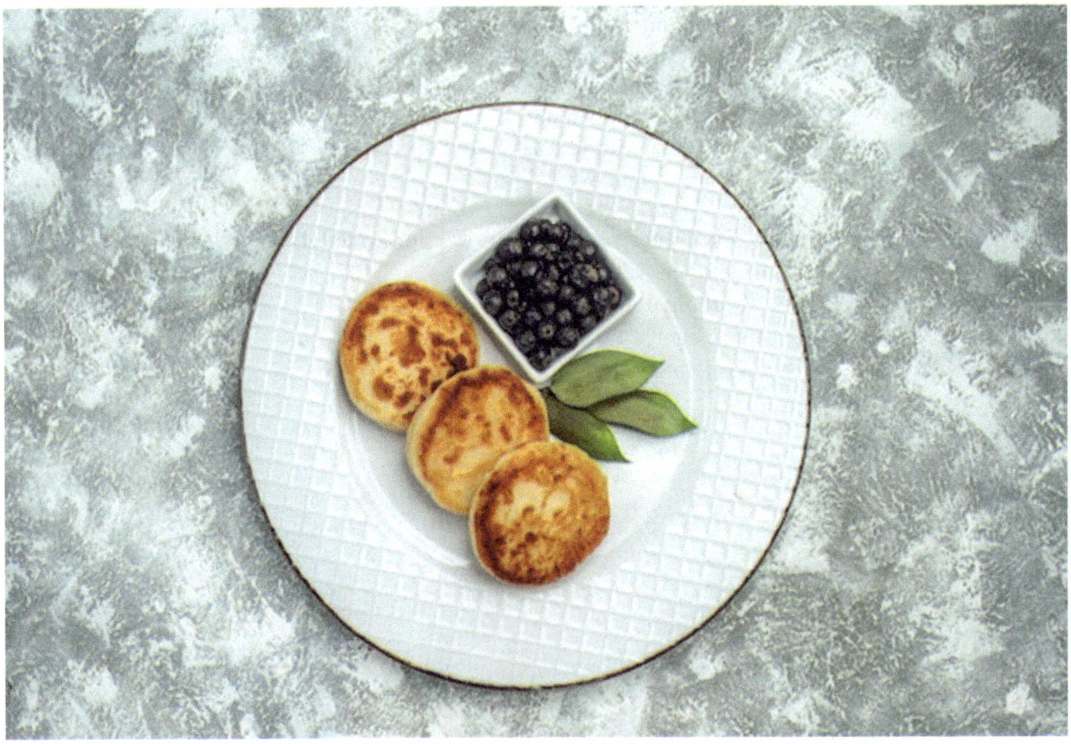

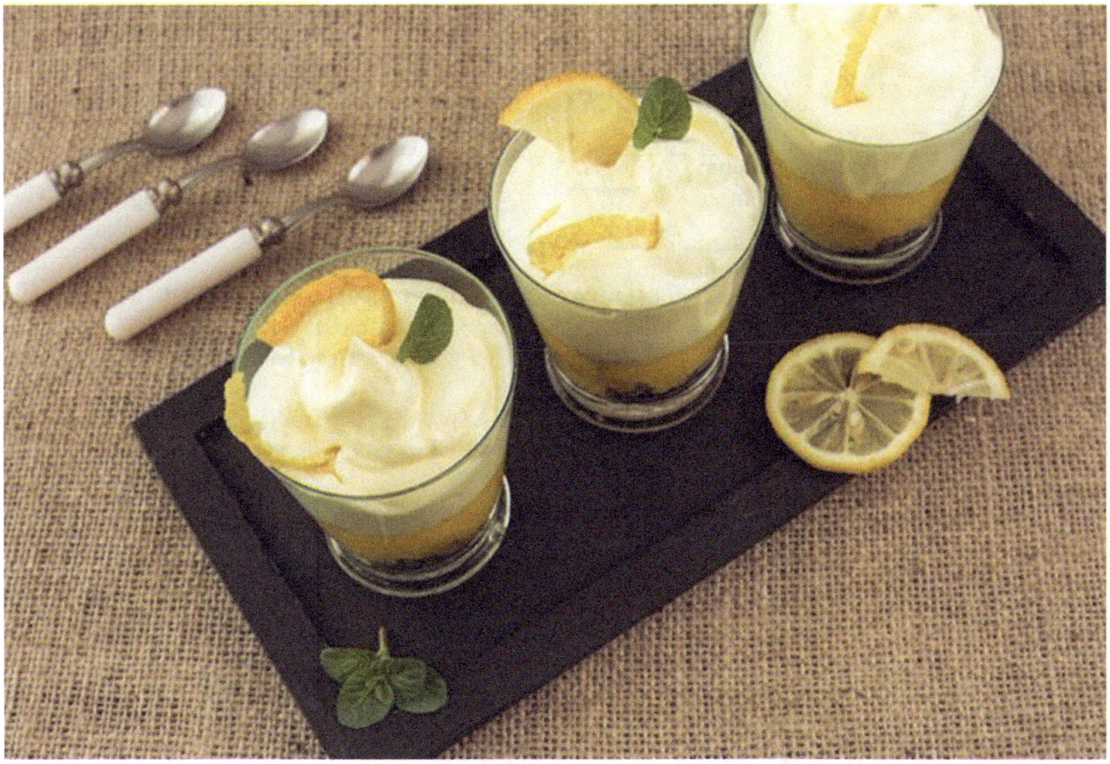

59. Sugar-Free Lemon Ginger Sorbet

Prep.Time: 15 min	**Cook Time:** 0 min	**Serving:** 4	**Beverage pairing:** Ginger Tea

Ingredients:

- 1 cup water
- 1/2 cup fresh lemon juice
- Zest of 1 lemon
- 1/4 cup grated ginger
- 1/4 cup sugar-free sweetener (erythritol or stevia)

Preparation:

1. In a saucepan, combine water, fresh lemon juice, lemon zest, grated ginger, and sugar-free sweetener.
2. Heat the mixture over medium heat until it starts to simmer, stirring to dissolve the sweetener.
3. Remove from heat and let it cool to room temperature.
4. Strain the mixture to remove ginger and lemon zest.
5. Pour the liquid into an ice cream maker and churn according to the manufacturer's instructions.
6. Transfer the sorbet to a lidded container and freeze for at least 4 hours before serving.

Nutrient Facts (per serving - serves approximately 4):

- Calories: 30
- Carbohydrates: 5g
- Fat: 0g
- Protein: 0g

60. Vanilla Coconut Flour Cupcakes

Prep.Time:	Cook Time:	Serving:	Beverage pairing:
10 min	20 min	6	Herbal Tea

Ingredients:

- 1/2 cup coconut flour
- 1/4 cup melted coconut oil
- 1/4 cup unsweetened coconut milk
- 4 large eggs
- 1/4 cup sugar-free sweetener (erythritol or stevia)
- 1 teaspoon vanilla extract
- 1/2 teaspoon baking powder
- A pinch of salt

Preparation:

1. Preheat the oven to 350°F (175°C) and line a cupcake tin with paper liners.
2. In a bowl, whisk together coconut flour, melted coconut oil, coconut milk, eggs, sugar-free sweetener, vanilla extract, baking powder, and a pinch of salt until well combined.
3. Spoon the batter into the cupcake liners, filling each about 2/3 full.
4. Bake for 18-20 minutes or until a toothpick inserted into the center comes out clean.
5. Allow the cupcakes to cool in the tin for 5 minutes before transferring them to a wire rack to cool completely.

Nutrient Facts (per cupcake - makes approximately 6):

- Calories: 100
- Carbohydrates: 5g
- Fat: 8g
- Protein: 3g

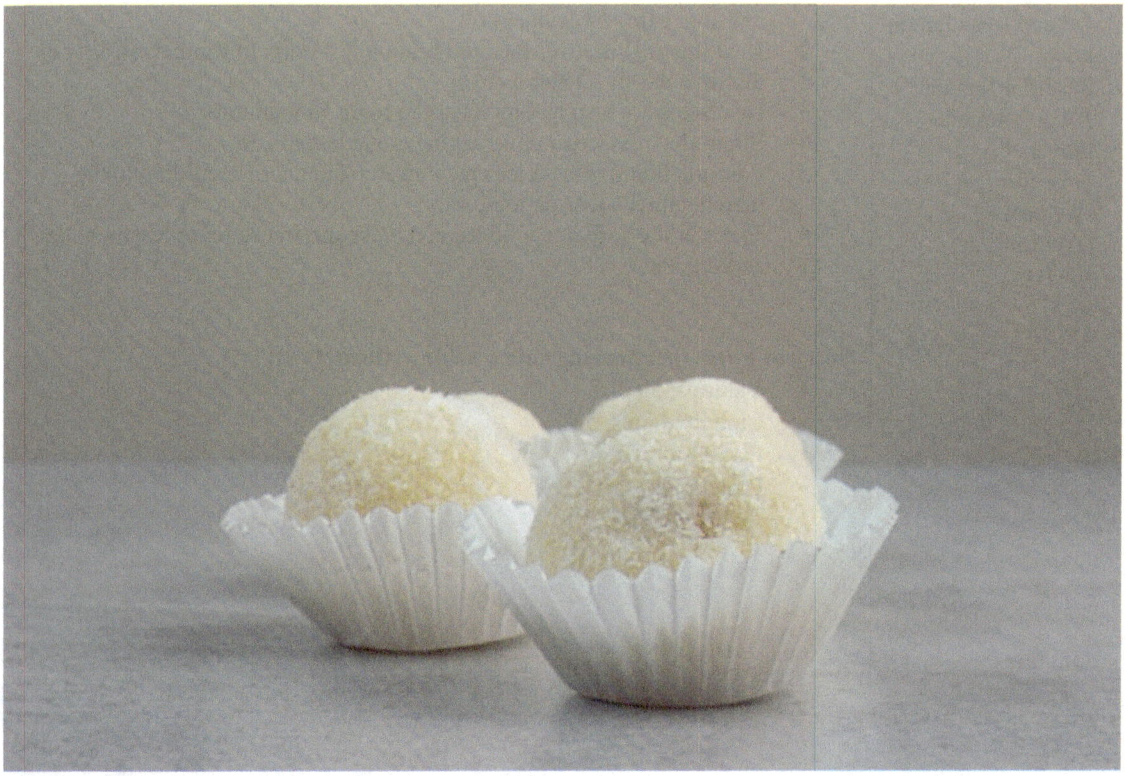

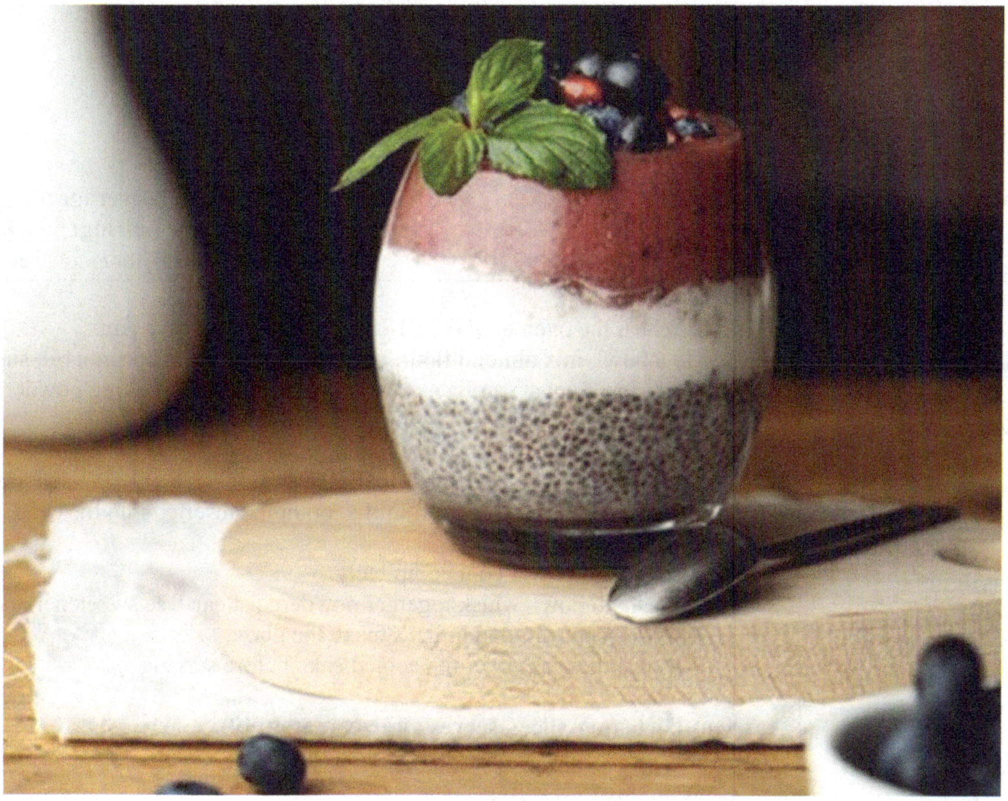

61. Chia Seed and Berry Parfait

Prep.Time: 5 min

Cook Time: 0 min

Serving: 2

Beverage pairing: Herbal Tea

Ingredients:

- 1/4 cup chia seeds
- 1 cup unsweetened almond milk
- Stevia to taste
- 1 cup mixed berries (strawberries, blueberries, raspberries)
- Sugar-free granola for layering

Preparation:

1. In a bowl, whisk together chia seeds, almond milk, and stevia.
2. Refrigerate the mixture for at least 2 hours or overnight, stirring occasionally.
3. Before serving, adjust sweetness with more stevia if needed.
4. In serving glasses, layer the chia pudding with mixed berries and sugar-free granola.

Nutrient Facts (per parfait - serves approximately 2):

- Calories: 150
- Carbohydrates: 15g
- Fat: 8g
- Protein: 4g

62. No-Sugar Added Apple Walnut Cake

Prep.Time: 15 min | **Cook Time:** 30 min | **Serving:** 10 | **Beverage pairing:** Cinnamon Tea

Ingredients:

- 2 cups almond flour
- 1/4 cup coconut flour
- 1/2 cup melted coconut oil
- 1/2 cup sugar-free sweetener (erythritol or stevia)
- 4 large eggs
- 1 teaspoon vanilla extract
- 1 teaspoon ground cinnamon
- 1/2 teaspoon baking powder
- A pinch of salt
- 1 cup grated apples (with skin)
- 1/2 cup chopped walnuts

Preparation:

1. Preheat the oven to 350°F (175°C) and grease a cake pan.
2. In a bowl, mix almond flour, coconut flour, melted coconut oil, sugar-free sweetener, eggs, vanilla extract, ground cinnamon, baking powder, and a pinch of salt until well combined.
3. Fold in grated apples and chopped walnuts.
4. Pour the batter into the prepared cake pan.
5. Bake for 30-35 minutes or until a toothpick inserted into the center comes out clean.
6. Allow the cake to cool completely.
7. In a small bowl, whisk together powdered sugar-free sweetener and unsweetened almond milk to make the glaze.
8. Drizzle the glaze over the cooled cake before serving.

Nutrient Facts (per slice - serves approximately 10):

- Calories: 180
- Carbohydrates: 10g
- Fat: 15g
- Protein: 5g

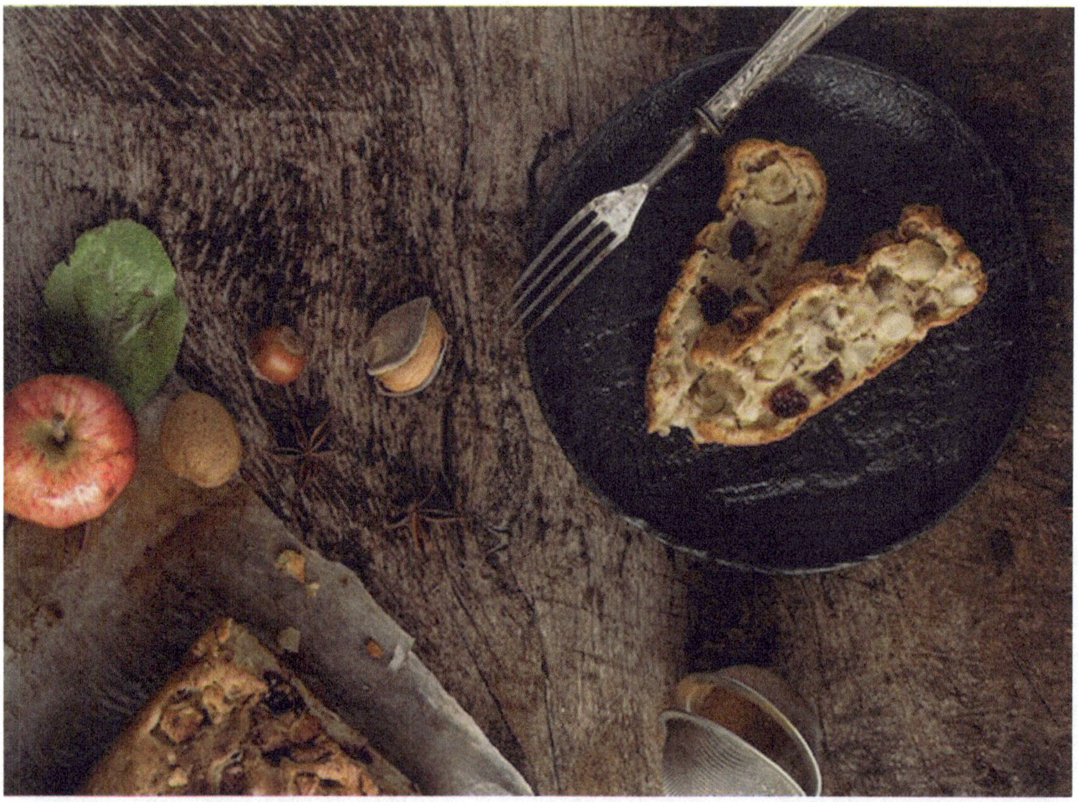

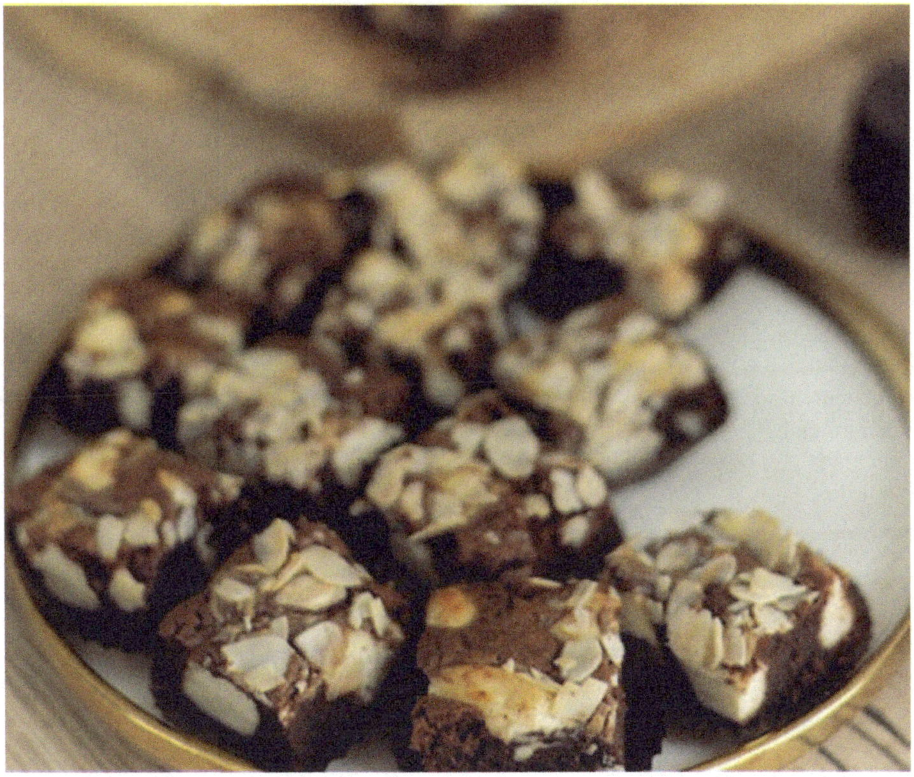

63. Almond Butter Chocolate Protein Bites

Prep.Time: 15 min

Cook Time: 0 min

Serving: 12

Beverage pairing: Black Coffee

Ingredients:

- 1 cup almond butter (unsweetened)
- 1/4 cup protein powder (chocolate-flavored)
- 1/4 cup unsweetened cocoa powder
- 2 tablespoons melted coconut oil
- Stevia to taste
- Shredded coconut for coating (optional)

Preparation:

1. In a bowl, mix almond butter, chocolate-flavored protein powder, unsweetened cocoa powder, melted coconut oil, and stevia until well combined.
2. Adjust sweetness with more stevia if needed.
3. Roll the mixture into bite-sized balls.
4. Optional: Roll each ball in shredded coconut for coating.
5. Refrigerate for at least 1 hour before serving.

Nutrient Facts (per protein bite - makes approximately 12):

- Calories: 100
- Carbohydrates: 4g
- Fat: 8g
- Protein: 4g

64. Cinnamon Roasted Pecans

Prep.Time:	Cook Time:	Serving:	Beverage pairing:
5 min	12 min	4	Cinnamon Coffee

Ingredients:

- 1 cup pecan halves
- 1 tablespoon melted coconut oil
- 1 teaspoon ground cinnamon
- Stevia to taste

Preparation:

1. Preheat the oven to 325°F (163°C) and line a baking sheet with parchment paper.
2. In a bowl, toss pecan halves with melted coconut oil, ground cinnamon, and stevia.
3. Spread the pecans in a single layer on the prepared baking sheet.
4. Roast for 10-12 minutes or until fragrant, stirring halfway through.
5. Allow the cinnamon roasted pecans to cool completely before serving.

Nutrient Facts (per serving - makes approximately 1 cup):

- Calories: 120
- Carbohydrates: 4g
- Fat: 12g
- Protein: 2g

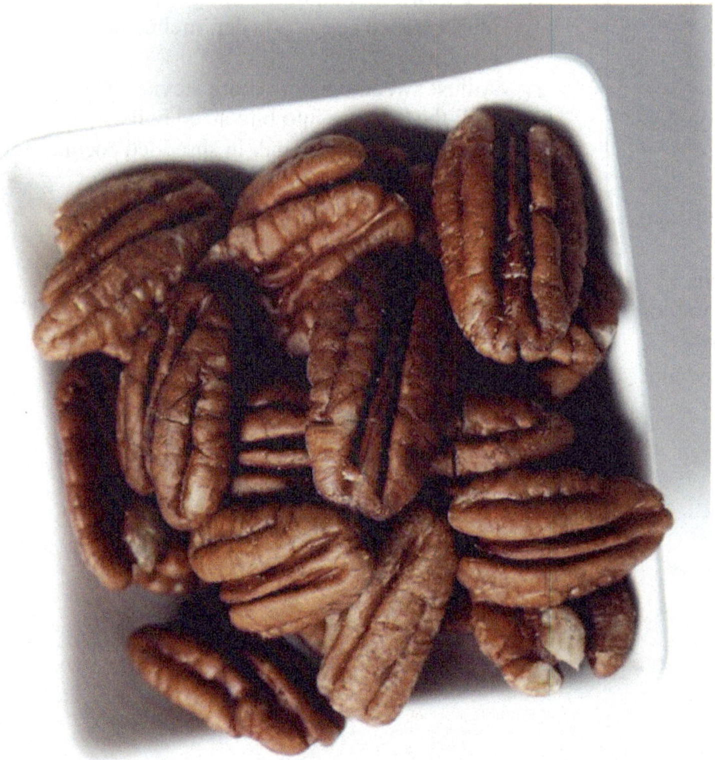

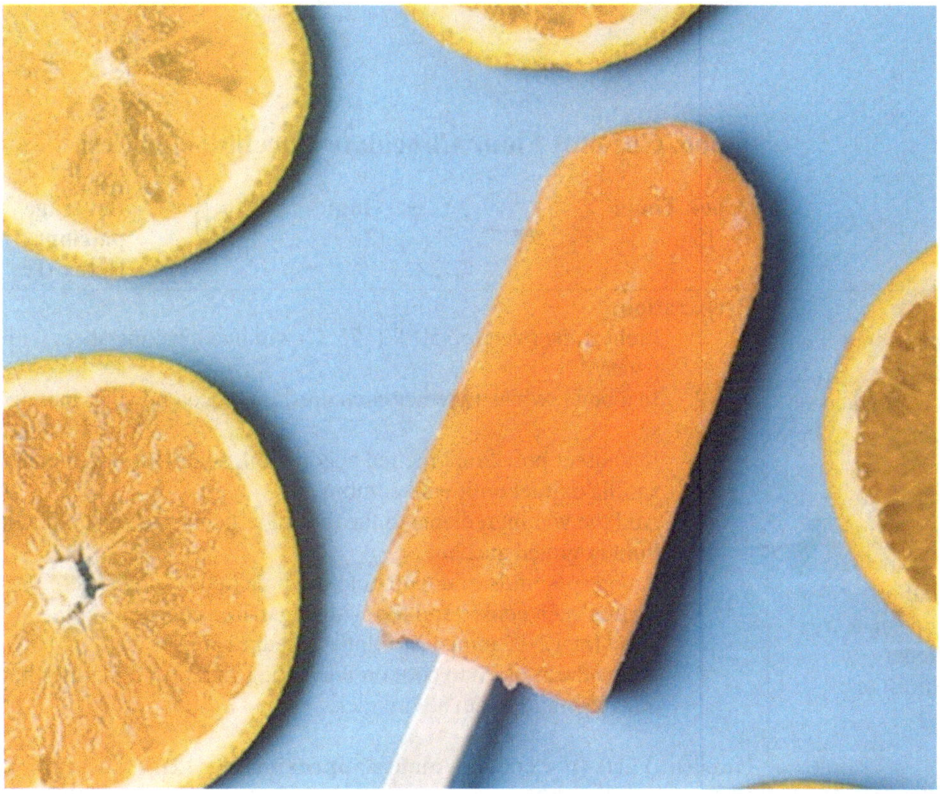

65. Sugar-Free Orange Creamsicles

Prep.Time: 10 min

Cook Time: 0 min

Serving: 6

Beverage pairing: Orange Juice

Ingredients:

- 1 cup fresh orange juice
- 1 cup unsweetened coconut milk
- 1 teaspoon vanilla extract
- Stevia to taste

Preparation:

1. In a bowl, whisk together fresh orange juice, unsweetened coconut milk, vanilla extract, and stevia.
2. Adjust sweetness with more stevia if needed.
3. Pour the mixture into popsicle molds.
4. Freeze for at least 4 hours or until fully set.
5. Run the molds under warm water to release the creamsicles before serving.

Nutrient Facts (per creamsicle - makes approximately 6):

- Calories: 50
- Carbohydrates: 4g
- Fat: 4g
- Protein: 1g

66. Coconut Flour Chocolate Zucchini Cookies

Prep.Time: 15 min	Cook Time: 15 min	Serving: 12	Beverage pairing: Herbal Tea

Ingredients:

- 1 cup coconut flour
- 1/2 cup unsweetened cocoa powder
- 1/2 teaspoon baking soda
- 1/4 teaspoon salt
- 1/2 cup melted coconut oil
- 1/2 cup sugar-free sweetener (erythritol or stevia)
- 3 large eggs
- 1 teaspoon vanilla extract
- 1 cup grated zucchini
- Sugar-free chocolate chips for topping

Preparation:

1. Preheat the oven to 350°F (175°C) and line a baking sheet with parchment paper.
2. In a bowl, whisk together coconut flour, cocoa powder, baking soda, and salt.
3. In another bowl, mix melted coconut oil, sugar-free sweetener, eggs, and vanilla extract until well combined.
4. Add the wet ingredients to the dry ingredients and stir until a dough forms.
5. Fold in grated zucchini.
6. Scoop spoonfuls of dough onto the prepared baking sheet.
7. Flatten each cookie and top with sugar-free chocolate chips.
8. Bake for 12-15 minutes or until the edges are set.
9. Allow the cookies to cool on the baking sheet for 5 minutes before transferring them to a wire rack.

Nutrient Facts (per cookie - makes approximately 12):

- Calories: 120
- Carbohydrates: 8g
- Fat: 9g
- Protein: 3g

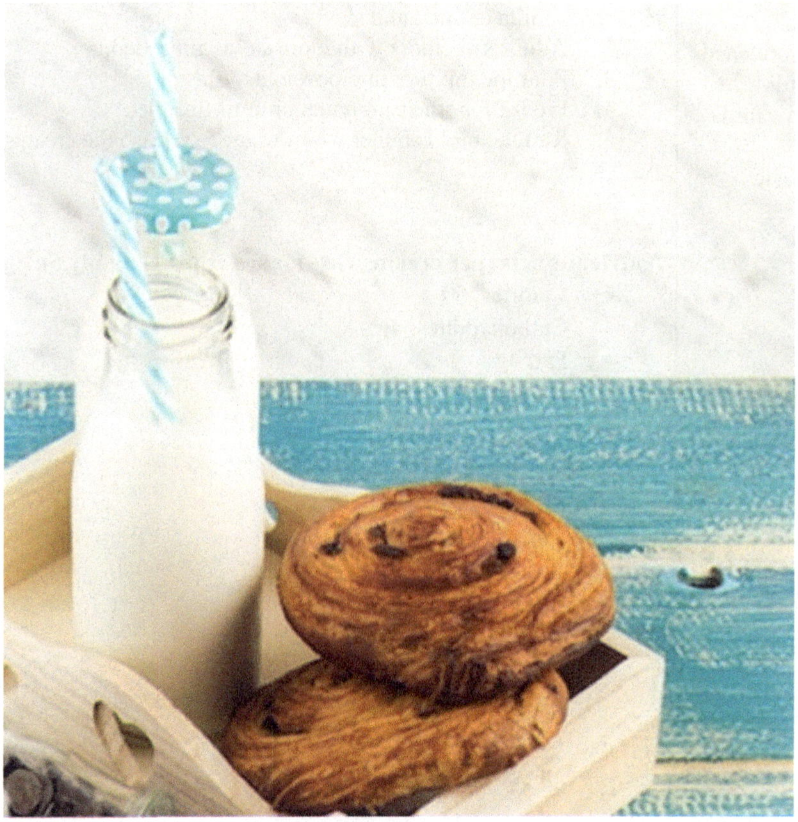

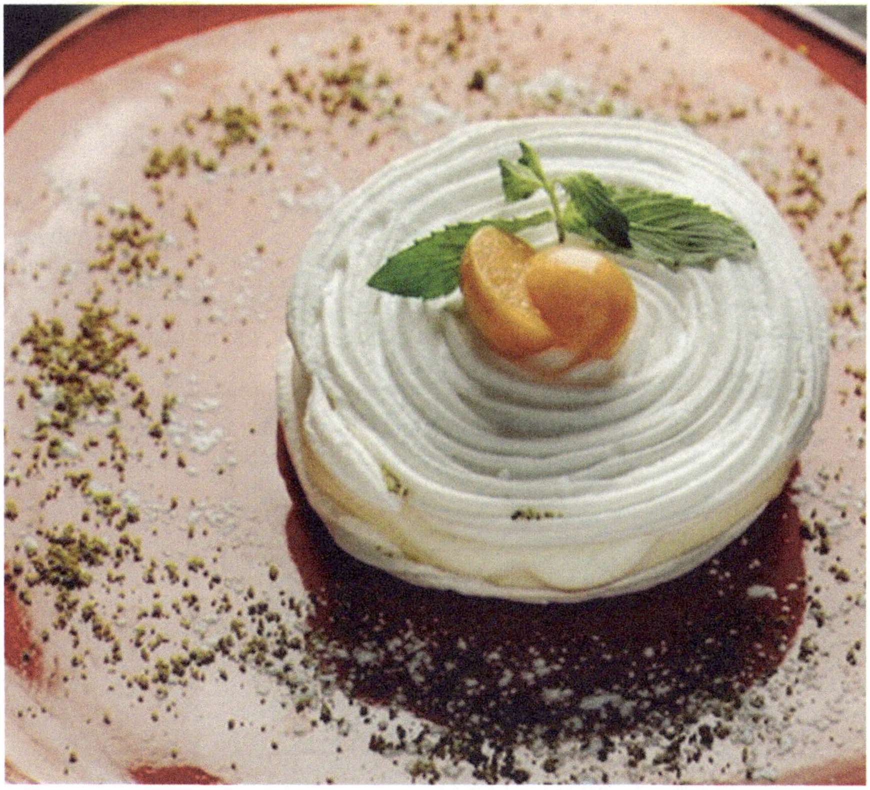

67. Vanilla Almond Milk Panna Cotta

Prep.Time: 10 min

Cook Time: 0 min

Serving: 4

Beverage pairing: Chamamile Tea

Ingredients:

- 2 cups unsweetened almond milk
- 1 teaspoon vanilla extract
- 1/4 cup sugar-free sweetener (erythritol or stevia)
- 2 tablespoons cold water
- 1 1/2 teaspoons gelatin

Preparation:

1. In a saucepan, heat almond milk, vanilla extract, and sugar-free sweetener over medium heat until it starts to simmer.
2. In a small bowl, mix cold water and gelatin. Let it sit for a minute to bloom.
3. Add the bloomed gelatin to the saucepan and whisk until fully dissolved.
4. Remove from heat and let it cool to room temperature.
5. Pour the mixture into serving glasses.
6. Refrigerate for at least 4 hours or until set.

Nutrient Facts (per serving - serves approximately 4):

- Calories: 50
- Carbohydrates: 1g
- Fat: 4g
- Protein: 1g

68. Pumpkin Pie Greek Yogurt Bowl

Prep.Time:	Cook Time:	Serving:	Beverage pairing:
5 min	0 min	1	Herbal Tea

Ingredients:

- 1 cup plain Greek yogurt
- 1/4 cup pumpkin puree
- 1/2 teaspoon pumpkin pie spice
- Stevia to taste
- Chopped pecans for topping

Preparation:

1. In a bowl, mix plain Greek yogurt, pumpkin puree, pumpkin pie spice, and stevia until well combined.
2. Adjust sweetness with more stevia if needed.
3. Spoon the pumpkin pie Greek yogurt into a serving bowl.
4. Top with chopped pecans before serving.

Nutrient Facts (per bowl - serves 1):

- Calories: 200
- Carbohydrates: 10g
- Fat: 15g
- Protein: 15g

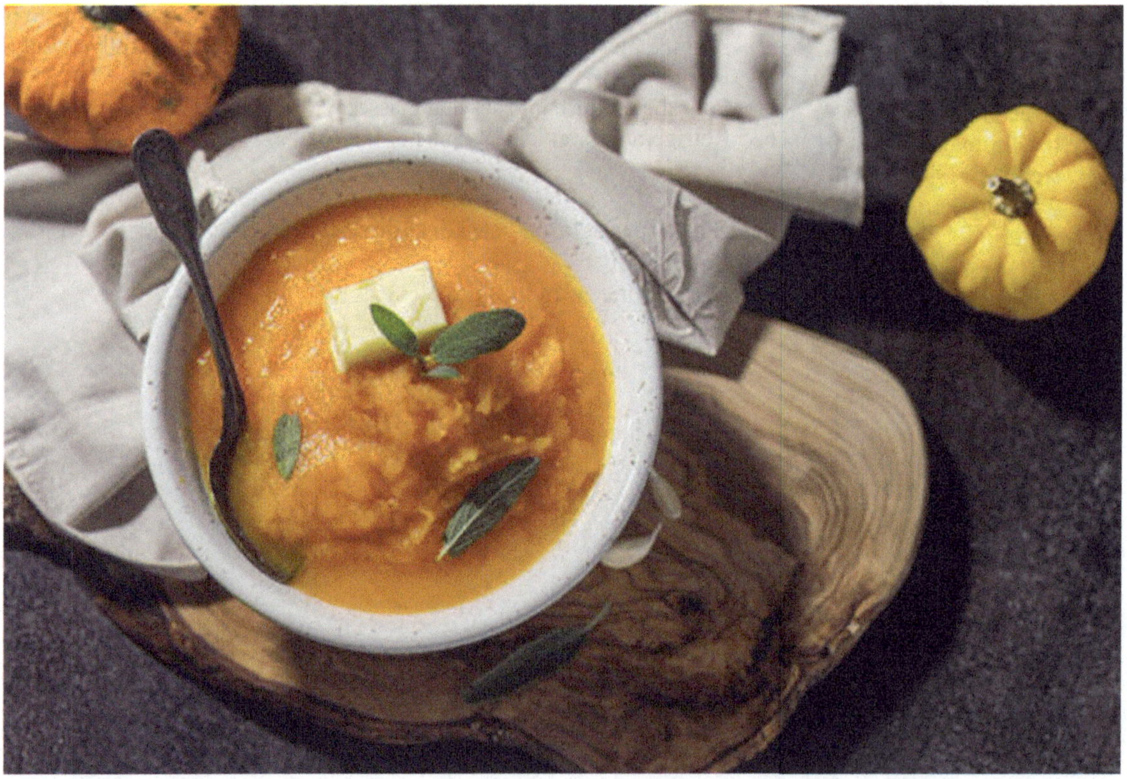

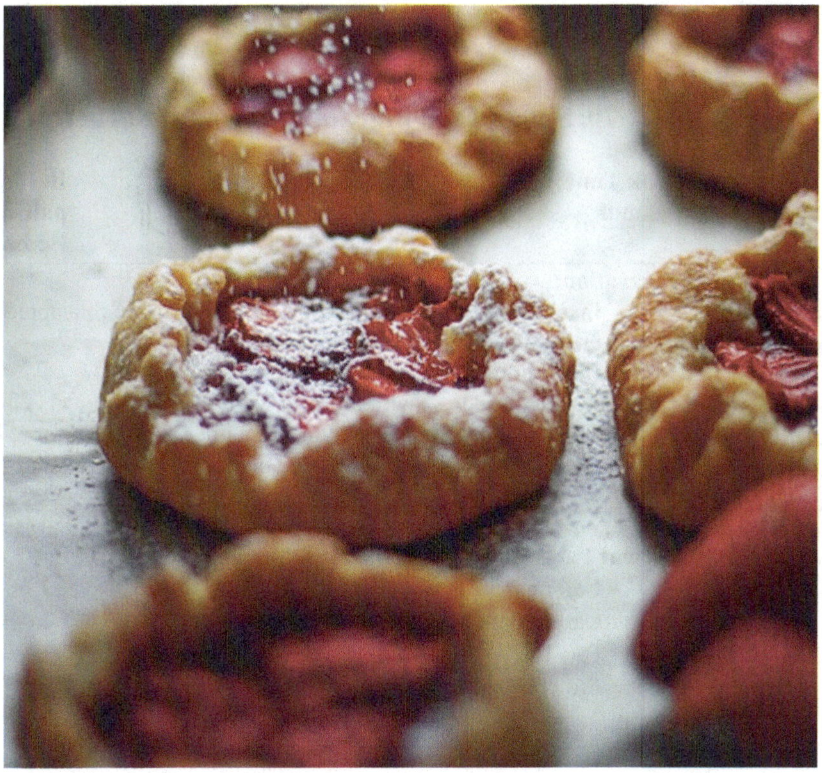

69. Raspberry Almond Flour Scones

Prep.Time: 15 min

Cook Time: 25 min

Serving: 8

Beverage pairing: BlackTea

Ingredients:

- 2 cups almond flour
- 1/4 cup coconut flour
- 1/4 cup melted coconut oil
- 1/4 cup sugar-free sweetener (erythritol or stevia)
- 2 large eggs
- 1 teaspoon almond extract
- 1/2 teaspoon baking powder
- A pinch of salt
- 1/2 cup fresh raspberries

Preparation:

1. Preheat the oven to 350°F (175°C) and line a baking sheet with parchment paper.
2. In a bowl, mix almond flour, coconut flour, melted coconut oil, sugar-free sweetener, eggs, almond extract, baking powder, and a pinch of salt until well combined.
3. Gently fold in fresh raspberries.
4. Form the dough into a circle on the prepared baking sheet.
5. Cut the circle into 8 wedges.
6. Bake for 20-25 minutes or until the edges are golden brown.
7. Allow the scones to cool on the baking sheet for 5 minutes before transferring them to a wire rack.

Nutrient Facts (per scone - makes 8):

- Calories: 180
- Carbohydrates: 8g
- Fat: 15g
- Protein: 6g

70. Sugar-Free Pineapple Coconut Sorbet

Prep.Time:	Cook Time:	Serving:	Beverage pairing:
5 min	0 min	4	Herbal Tea

Ingredients:

- 2 cups frozen pineapple chunks
- 1/2 cup unsweetened coconut milk
- Stevia to taste
- Shredded coconut for garnish (optional)

Preparation:

1. In a blender or food processor, combine frozen pineapple chunks, unsweetened coconut milk, and stevia.
2. Blend until smooth and creamy.
3. Adjust sweetness with more stevia if needed.
4. Transfer the sorbet to a lidded container and freeze for at least 4 hours.
5. Garnish with shredded coconut before serving if desired.

Nutrient Facts (per serving - serves approximately 4):

- Calories: 50
- Carbohydrates: 12g
- Fat: 1g
- Protein: 0g

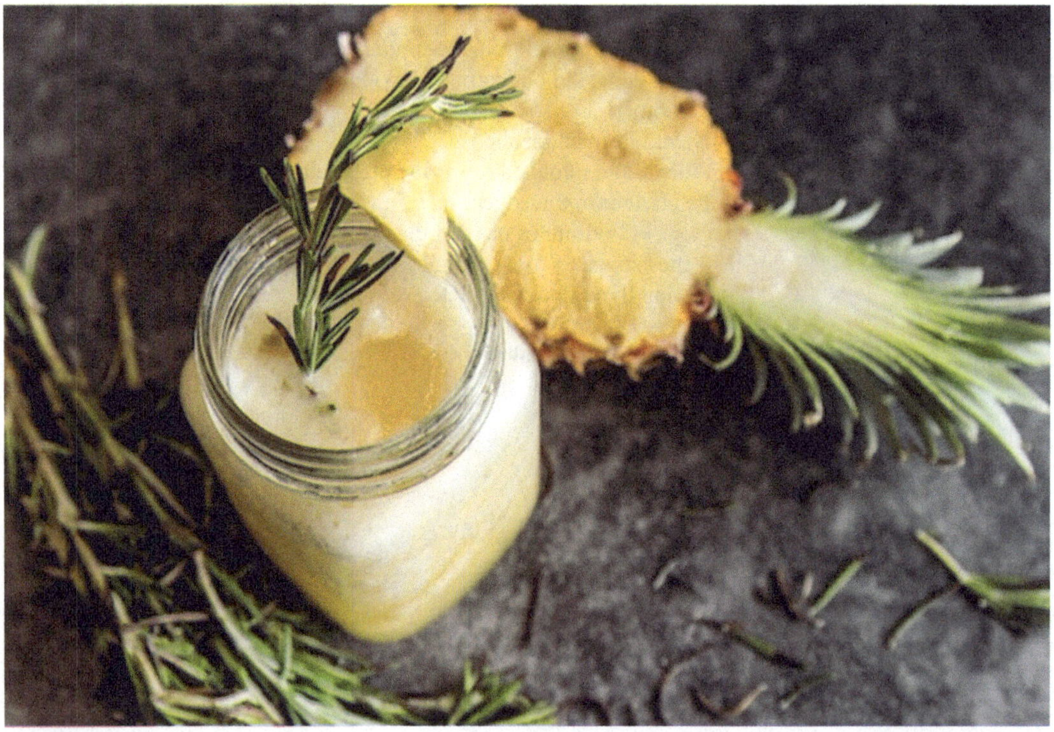

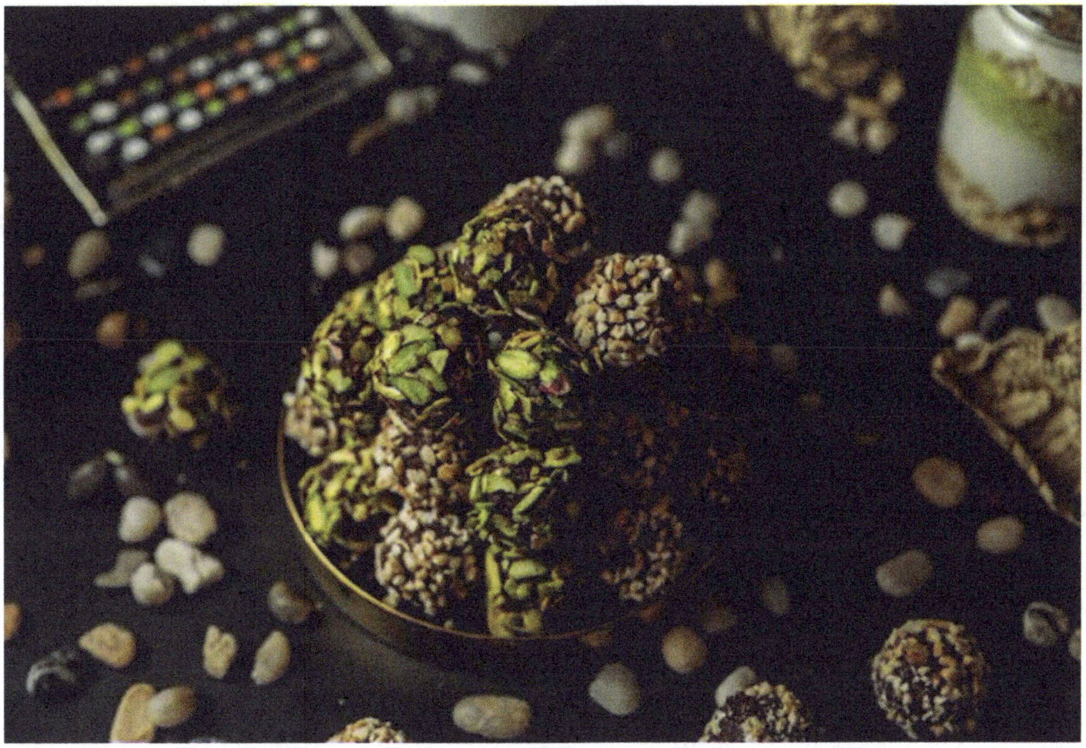

71. Dark Chocolate Avocado Truffles

Prep.Time: 15 min	Cook Time: 0 min	Serving: 12	Beverage pairing: Black Tea

Ingredients:

- 1 ripe avocado
- 1/2 cup dark chocolate chips (sugar-free or at least 70% cocoa)
- 2 tablespoons unsweetened cocoa powder
- 1 teaspoon vanilla extract
- Stevia to taste
- Pinch of salt
- Chopped nuts or shredded coconut for coating (optional)

Preparation:

1. In a blender or food processor, blend the avocado until smooth.
2. In a microwave-safe bowl, melt dark chocolate chips in 30-second intervals, stirring between each interval until smooth.
3. Add melted chocolate, unsweetened cocoa powder, vanilla extract, stevia, and a pinch of salt to the blended avocado. Blend until well combined.
4. Refrigerate the mixture for at least 2 hours or until firm.
5. Scoop spoonfuls of the mixture and roll them into truffle-sized balls.
6. Optional: Roll each truffle in chopped nuts or shredded coconut for coating.
7. Refrigerate for an additional 30 minutes before serving.

Nutrient Facts (per truffle - makes approximately 12):

- Calories: 60
- Carbohydrates: 4g
- Fat: 5g
- Protein: 1g

72. No-Bake Almond Joy Bars

Prep.Time:	Cook Time:	Serving:	Beverage pairing:
15 min	0 min	8	Herbal Tea

Ingredients:

- 1 cup almond flour
- 1/4 cup melted coconut oil
- 1/4 cup sugar-free sweetener (erythritol or stevia)
- 1/2 teaspoon almond extract
- A pinch of salt
- 1/2 cup unsweetened shredded coconut
- 1/4 cup melted coconut oil
- 1/4 cup dark chocolate chips (sugar-free or at least 70% cocoa)

Preparation:

1. In a bowl, mix almond flour, melted coconut oil, sugar-free sweetener, almond extract, and a pinch of salt to form the base.
2. Press the base mixture into a lined pan.
3. In another bowl, mix shredded coconut, melted coconut oil, and dark chocolate chips to create the topping.
4. Spread the topping over the base.
5. Refrigerate for at least 2 hours or until set.
6. Cut into bars before serving.

Nutrient Facts (per bar - makes approximately 8):

- Calories: 180
- Carbohydrates: 7g
- Fat: 16g
- Protein: 3g

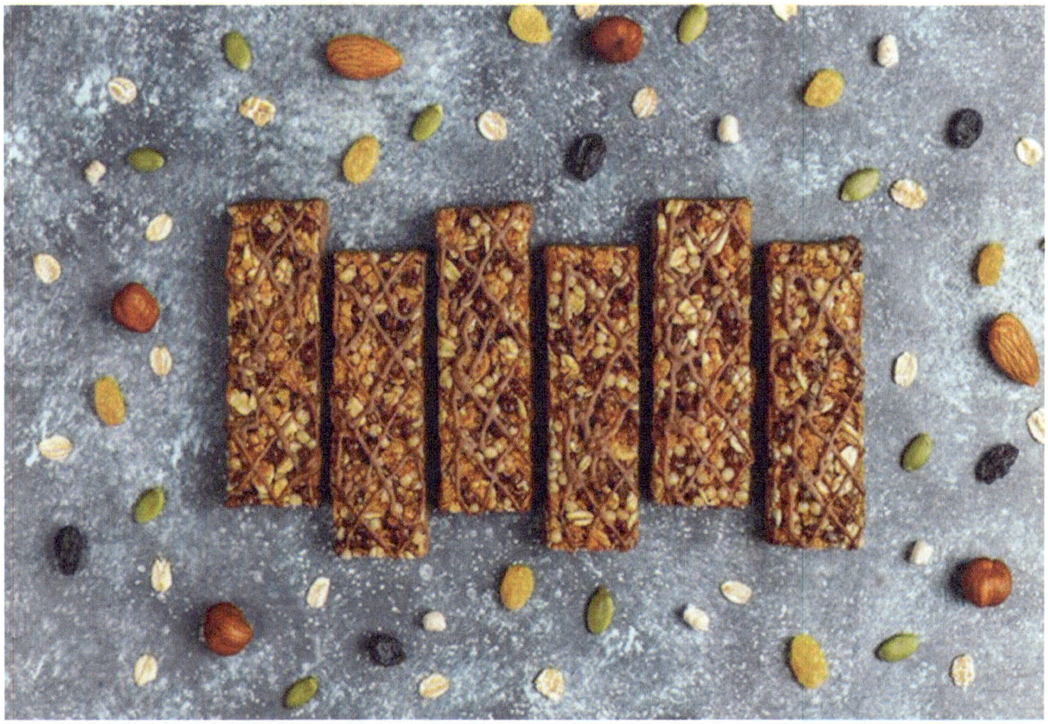

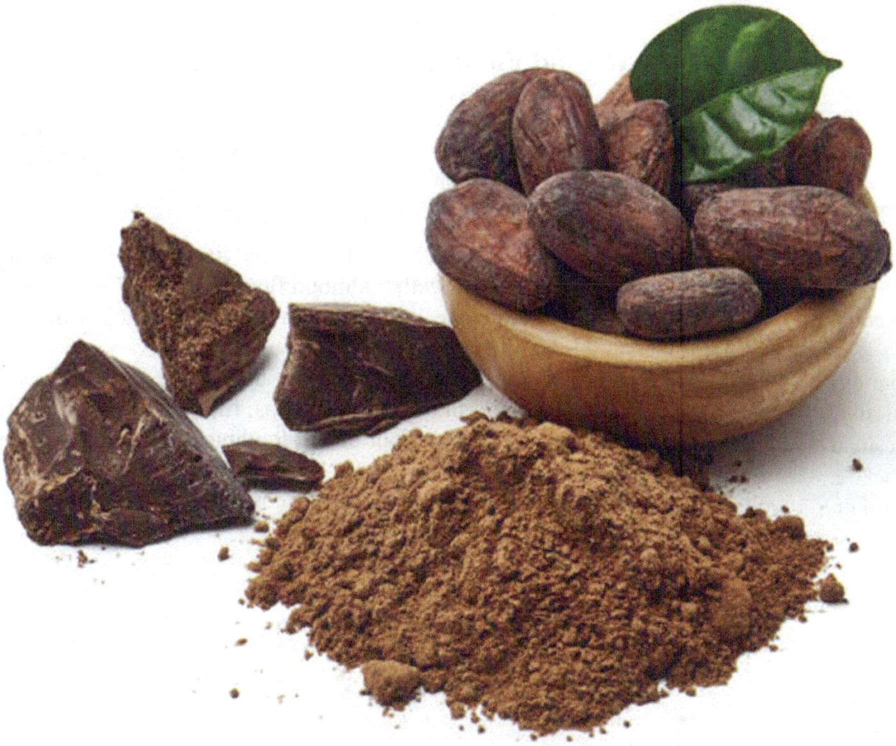

73. Cocoa-Dusted Cashews

Prep.Time:	Cook Time:	Serving:	Beverage pairing:
10 min	10 min	4	Tea

Ingredients:

- 1 cup raw cashews
- 2 tablespoons unsweetened cocoa powder
- Stevia to taste
- Pinch of salt

Preparation:

1. In a dry skillet over medium heat, toast cashews until they start to brown, about 5-7 minutes. Stir frequently to prevent burning.
2. In a bowl, toss toasted cashews with unsweetened cocoa powder, stevia, and a pinch of salt until well coated.
3. Allow the cocoa-dusted cashews to cool completely before serving.

Nutrient Facts (per serving - makes approximately 1 cup):

- Calories: 150
- Carbohydrates: 8g
- Fat: 12g
- Protein: 5g

74. Almond Flour Cranberry Orange Muffins

Prep.Time:	Cook Time:	Serving:	Beverage pairing:
10 min	20 min	12	Green Tea

Ingredients:

- 2 cups almond flour
- 1/4 cup coconut flour
- 1/4 cup melted coconut oil
- 1/4 cup sugar-free sweetener (erythritol or stevia)
- 3 large eggs
- 1 teaspoon vanilla extract
- 1/2 teaspoon baking powder
- A pinch of salt
- 1/2 cup fresh cranberries, chopped
- Zest of 1 orange

Preparation:

1. Preheat the oven to 350°F (175°C) and line a muffin tin with paper liners.
2. In a bowl, whisk together almond flour, coconut flour, melted coconut oil, sugar-free sweetener, eggs, vanilla extract, baking powder, and a pinch of salt until well combined.
3. Gently fold in chopped cranberries and orange zest.
4. Spoon the batter into the muffin cups, filling each about 2/3 full.
5. Bake for 20-25 minutes or until a toothpick inserted into the center comes out clean.
6. Allow the muffins to cool in the tin for 5 minutes before transferring them to a wire rack to cool completely.

Nutrient Facts (per muffin - makes approximately 12):

- Calories: 150
- Carbohydrates: 8g
- Fat: 12g
- Protein: 5g

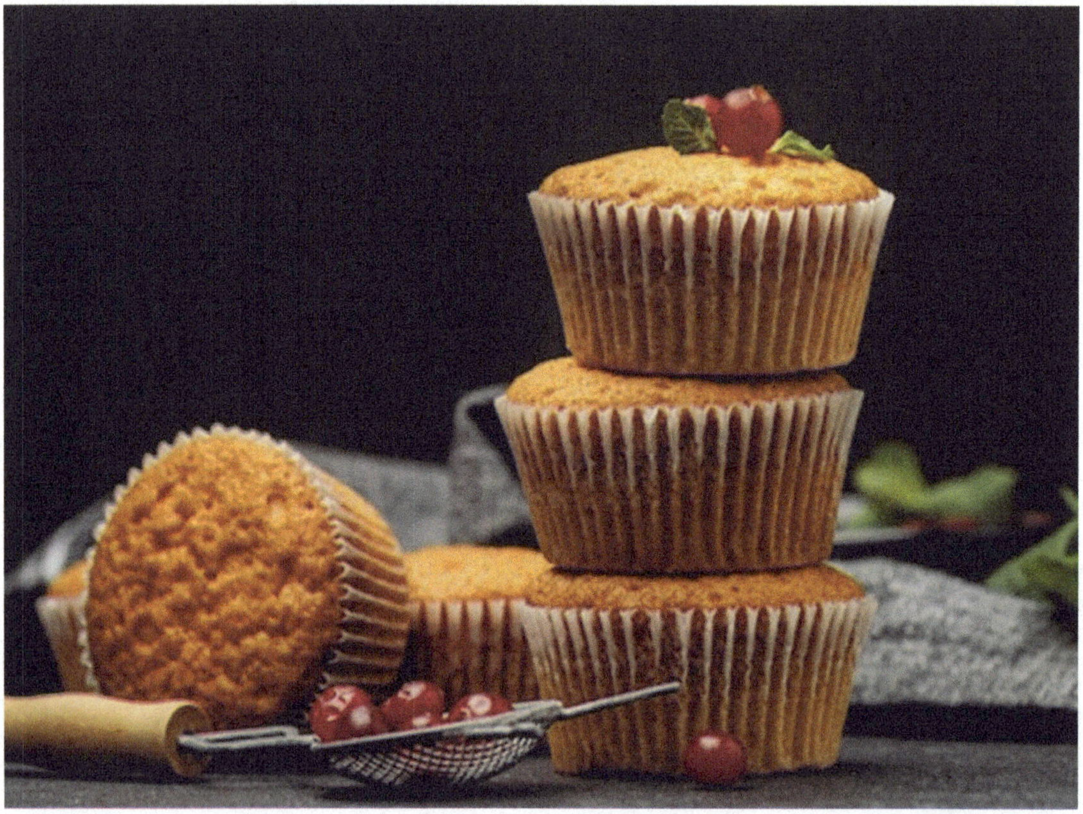

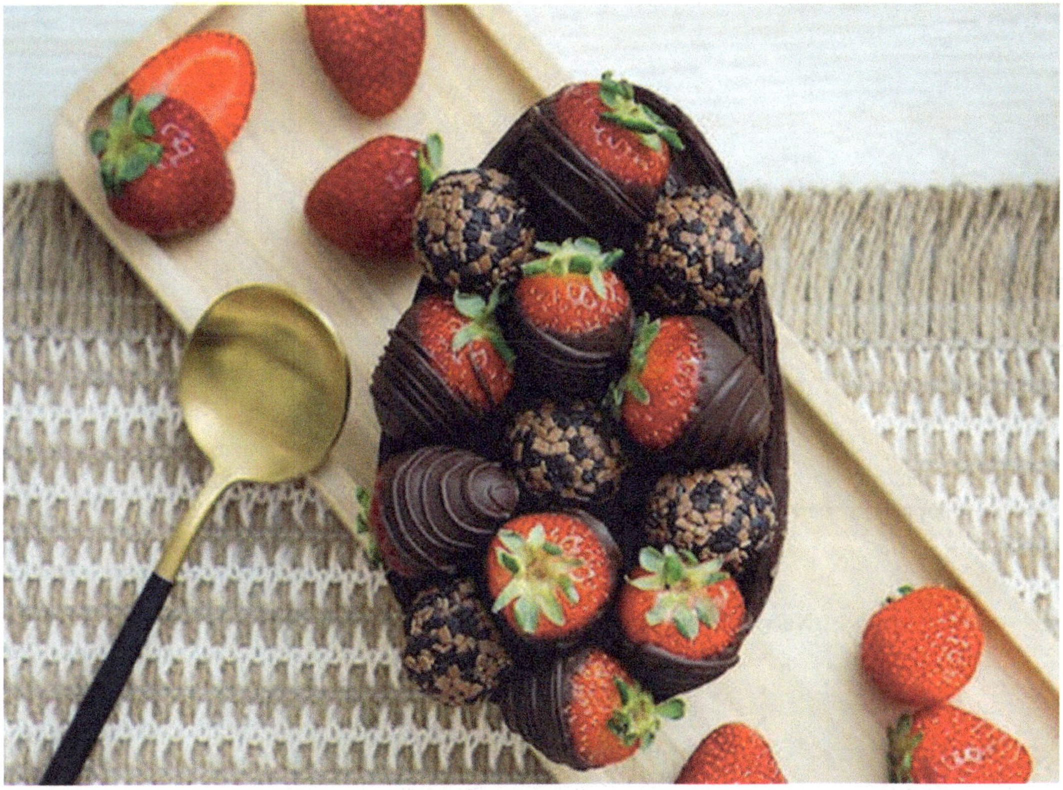

75. Greek Yogurt Chocolate Covered Strawberries

Prep.Time: 15 min

Cook Time: 30 min

Serving: 2

Beverage pairing: Herbal Tea

Ingredients:

- 1 cup plain Greek yogurt
- 1/4 cup unsweetened cocoa powder
- Stevia to taste
- 1 teaspoon vanilla extract
- 1 cup fresh strawberries, washed and dried

Preparation:

1. In a bowl, mix plain Greek yogurt, unsweetened cocoa powder, stevia, and vanilla extract until well combined.
2. Adjust sweetness with more stevia if needed.
3. Dip each strawberry into the chocolate yogurt mixture, coating them halfway.
4. Place the chocolate-covered strawberries on a parchment-lined tray.
5. Refrigerate for at least 30 minutes or until the chocolate is set.

Nutrient Facts (per serving - serves approximately 2):

- Calories: 100
- Carbohydrates: 12g
- Fat: 4g
- Protein: 8g

76. Pistachio Chia Seed Pudding

Prep.Time:	Cook Time:	Serving:	Beverage pairing:
5 min	0 min	2	Green Tea

Ingredients:

- 1/4 cup chia seeds
- 1 cup unsweetened almond milk
- Stevia to taste
- 1/4 teaspoon almond extract
- 1/4 cup chopped pistachios

Preparation:

1. In a bowl, whisk together chia seeds, almond milk, stevia, and almond extract.
2. Refrigerate the mixture for at least 2 hours or overnight, stirring occasionally.
3. Adjust sweetness with more stevia if needed.
4. Before serving, sprinkle chopped pistachios on top of the chia seed pudding.

Nutrient Facts (per serving - serves approximately 2):

- Calories: 200
- Carbohydrates: 15g
- Fat: 14g
- Protein: 6g

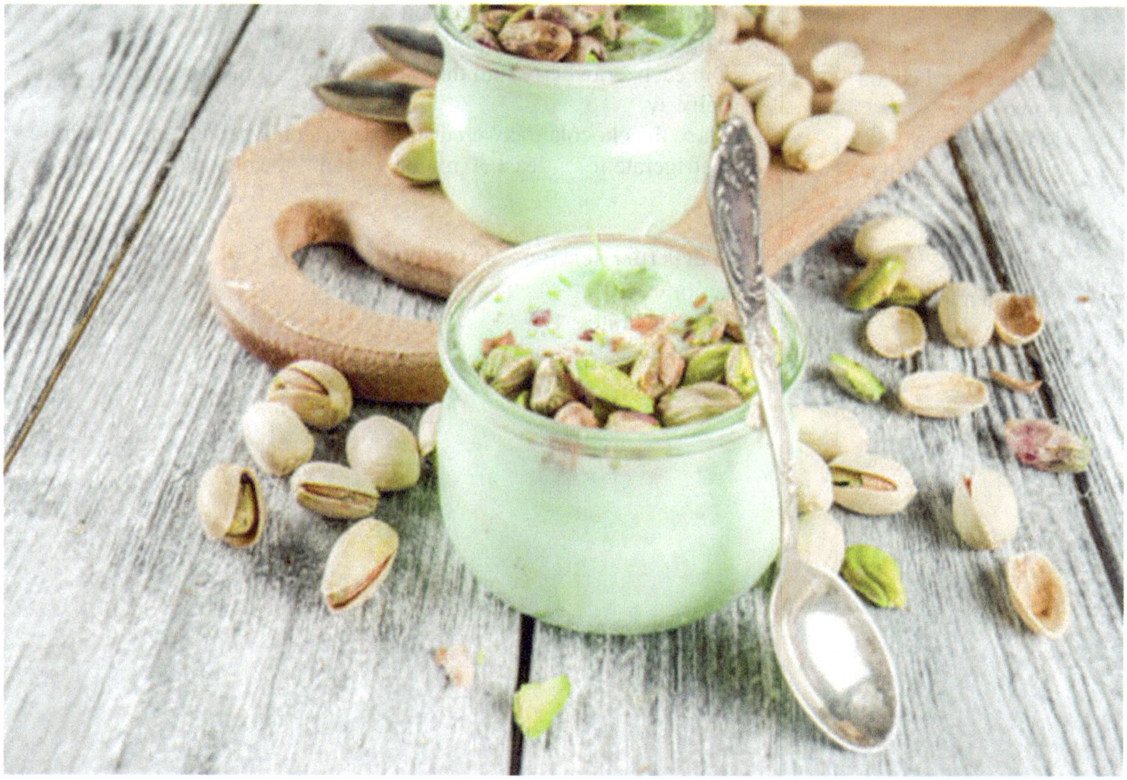

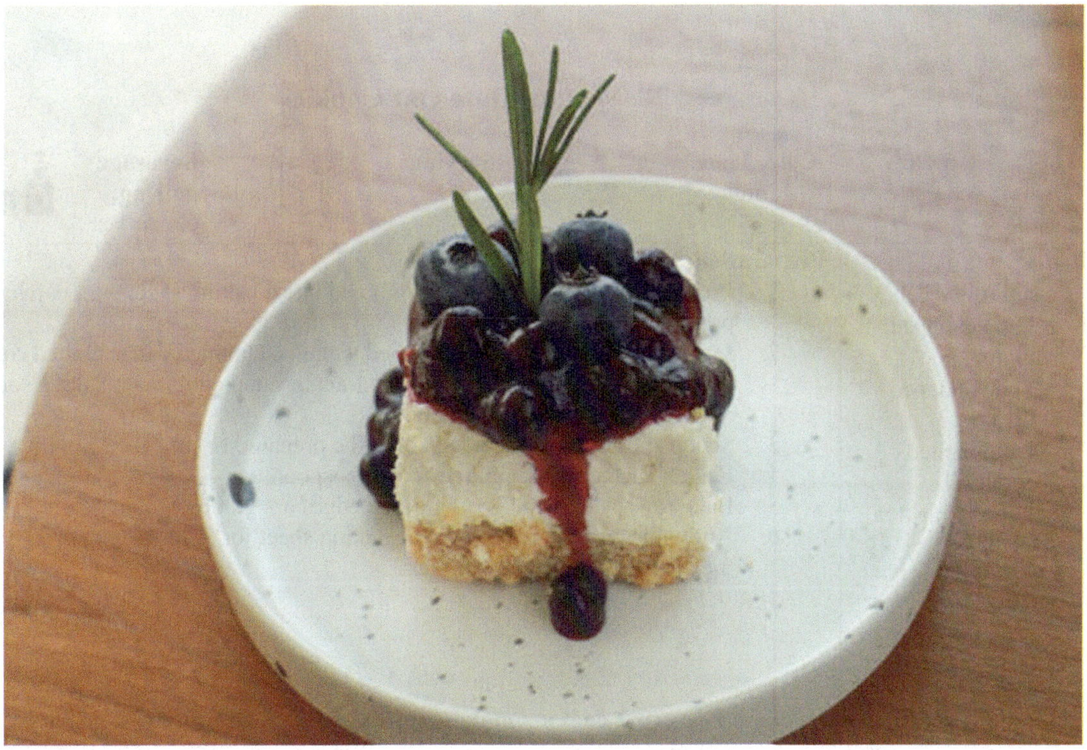

77. Sugar-Free Blueberry Cheesecake Bites

Prep.Time: 20 min | **Cook Time:** 0 min | **Serving:** 12 | **Beverage pairing:** Herbal Tea

Ingredients:

- 1 cup almond flour
- 1/4 cup melted coconut oil
- 1/4 cup sugar-free sweetener (erythritol or stevia)
- 1 cup cream cheese, softened
- 1/4 cup sugar-free sweetener
- 1 teaspoon vanilla extract
- Stevia to taste
- 1/2 cup fresh blueberries

Preparation:

1. In a bowl, mix almond flour, melted coconut oil, and sugar-free sweetener to form the crust.
2. Press the crust mixture into the bottom of a lined square pan.
3. In another bowl, beat together cream cheese, sugar-free sweetener, vanilla extract, and stevia until smooth.
4. Spread the cheesecake filling over the crust.
5. In a small saucepan, heat fresh blueberries with stevia until they release their juices.
6. Mash the blueberries and spread them over the cheesecake filling.
7. Refrigerate for at least 4 hours or until set.
8. Cut into bite-sized squares before serving.

Nutrient Facts (per cheesecake bite - makes approximately 12):

- Calories: 120
- Carbohydrates: 5g
- Fat: 10g
- Protein: 3g

78. Walnut Date Oat Cookies

Prep.Time: 15 min

Cook Time: 12 min

Serving: 12

Beverage pairing: Green Tea

Ingredients:

- 1 cup rolled oats
- 1/2 cup chopped walnuts
- 1/2 cup chopped dates
- 1/4 cup melted coconut oil
- 1/4 cup sugar-free sweetener (erythritol or stevia)
- 1 teaspoon vanilla extract
- 1/2 teaspoon ground cinnamon
- 1/4 teaspoon baking soda
- A pinch of salt

Preparation:

1. Preheat the oven to 350°F (175°C) and line a baking sheet with parchment paper.
2. In a bowl, mix rolled oats, chopped walnuts, chopped dates, melted coconut oil, sugar-free sweetener, vanilla extract, ground cinnamon, baking soda, and a pinch of salt until well combined.
3. Scoop spoonfuls of the dough onto the prepared baking sheet.
4. Flatten each cookie with the back of a spoon.
5. Bake for 10-12 minutes or until the edges are golden brown.
6. Allow the cookies to cool on the baking sheet for 5 minutes before transferring them to a wire rack.

Nutrient Facts (per cookie - makes approximately 12):

- Calories: 120
- Carbohydrates: 10g
- Fat: 8g
- Protein: 2g

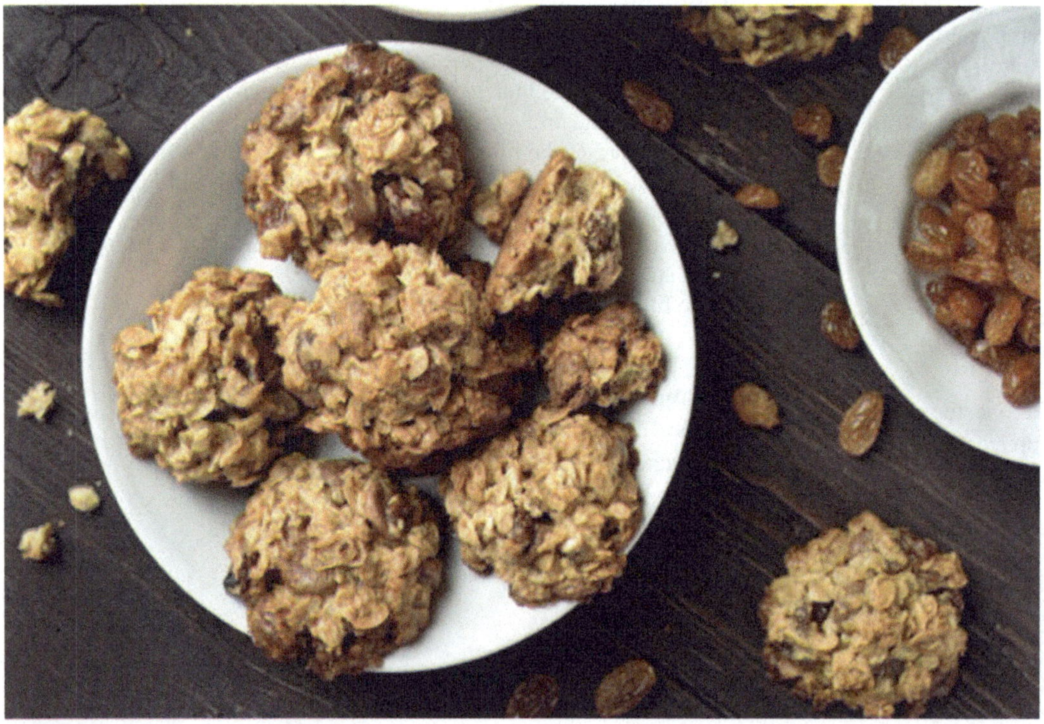

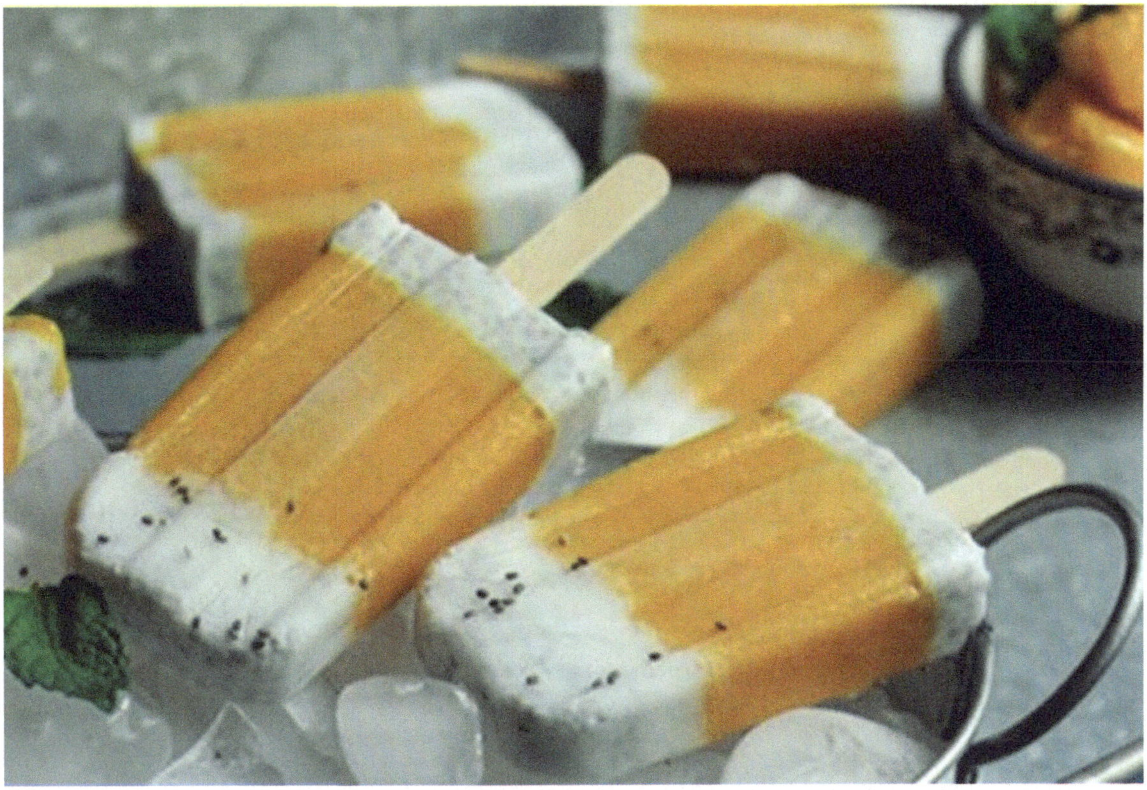

79. Mango Coconut Chia Seed Popsicles

Prep.Time:	Cook Time:	Serving:	Beverage pairing:
10 min	0 min	6	Green Tea

Ingredients:

- 1 cup ripe mango, diced
- 1 cup unsweetened coconut milk
- 2 tablespoons chia seeds
- Stevia to taste

Preparation:

1. In a blender, blend ripe mango until smooth.
2. In a bowl, mix mango puree, unsweetened coconut milk, chia seeds, and stevia until well combined.
3. Adjust sweetness with more stevia if needed.
4. Pour the mixture into popsicle molds.
5. Freeze for at least 4 hours or until fully set.
6. Run the molds under warm water to release the popsicles before serving.

Nutrient Facts (per popsicle - makes approximately 6):

- Calories: 50
- Carbohydrates: 8g
- Fat: 3g
- Protein: 1g

80. Cinnamon Vanilla Poached Pears

Prep.Time: 5 min

Cook Time: 20 min

Serving: 2

Beverage pairing: Herbal Tea

Ingredients:

- 2 ripe but firm pears, peeled and halved
- 2 cups water
- 1/4 cup sugar-free sweetener (erythritol or stevia)
- 1 cinnamon stick
- 1 teaspoon vanilla extract

Preparation:

1. In a saucepan, combine water, sugar-free sweetener, cinnamon stick, and vanilla extract.
2. Bring the mixture to a simmer over medium heat.
3. Add the peeled and halved pears to the simmering liquid.
4. Poach the pears for 15-20 minutes or until they are tender but not mushy.
5. Remove the pears from the liquid and let them cool.
6. Drizzle with the poaching liquid before serving.

Nutrient Facts (per serving - serves 2):

- Calories: 80
- Carbohydrates: 20g
- Fat: 0g
- Protein: 0g

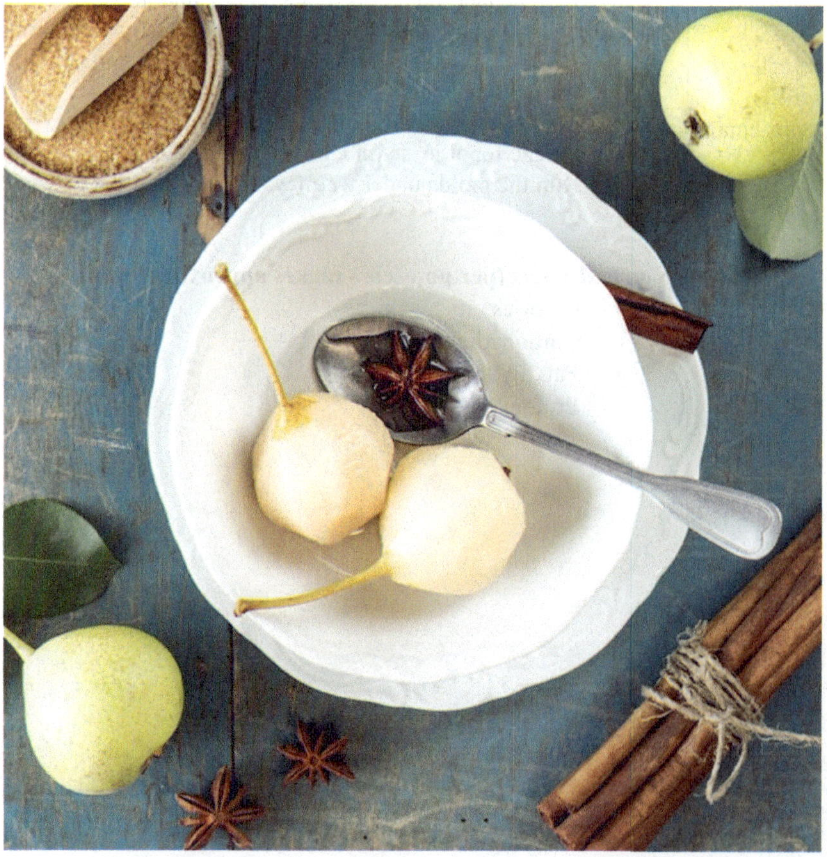

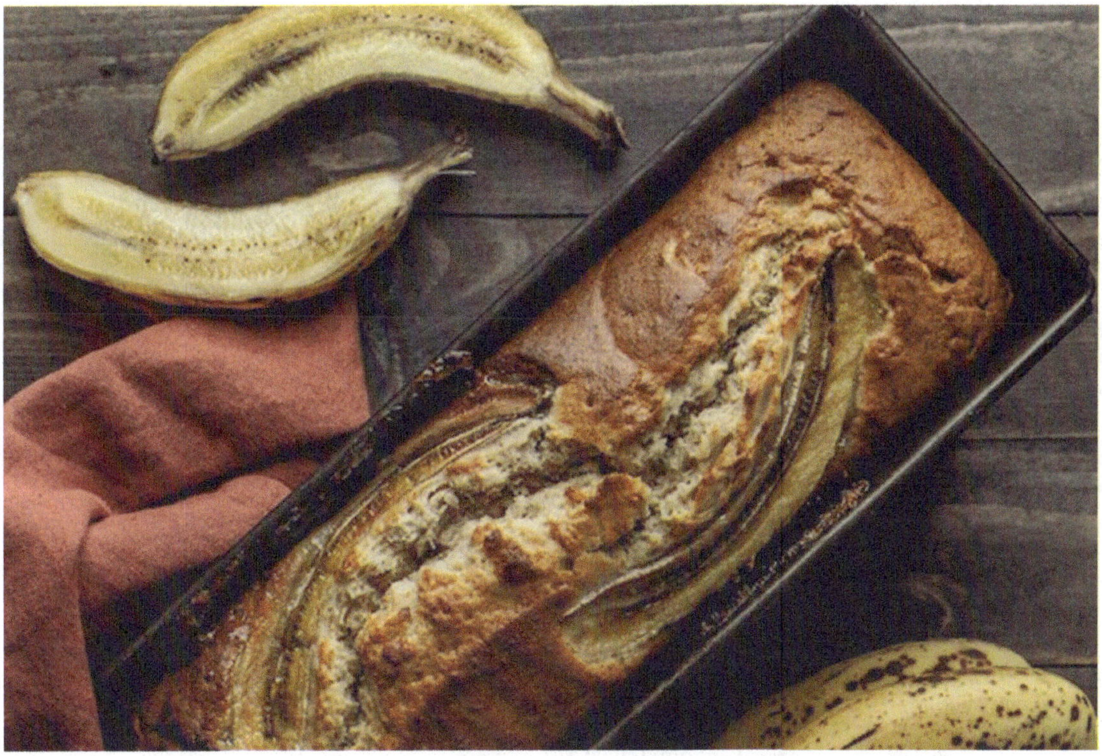

81. Chocolate Banana Bread

Prep.Time: 15 min

Cook Time: 45 min

Serving: 10

Beverage pairing: Black Tea

Ingredients:

- 2 ripe bananas, mashed
- 1 ripe avocado, mashed
- 1/4 cup melted coconut oil
- 1/4 cup sugar-free sweetener (erythritol or stevia)
- 2 large eggs
- 1 teaspoon vanilla extract
- 1 1/2 cups almond flour
- 1/4 cup cocoa powder
- 1/2 teaspoon baking soda
- 1/4 teaspoon salt
- Sugar-free chocolate chips for topping

Preparation:

1. Preheat the oven to 350°F (175°C) and grease a loaf pan.
2. In a bowl, mix mashed bananas, mashed avocado, melted coconut oil, sugar-free sweetener, eggs, and vanilla extract until well combined.
3. In another bowl, whisk together almond flour, cocoa powder, baking soda, and salt.
4. Combine the wet and dry ingredients until just combined.
5. Pour the batter into the prepared loaf pan.
6. Sprinkle sugar-free chocolate chips on top.
7. Bake for 40-45 minutes or until a toothpick inserted into the center comes out clean.
8. Allow the banana bread to cool in the pan for 10 minutes before transferring it to a wire rack.

Nutrient Facts (per slice - serves approximately 10):

- Calories: 150
- Carbohydrates: 12g
- Fat: 10g
- Protein: 4g

82. No-Sugar Added Lemon Coconut Bars

Prep.Time: 15 min	Cook Time: 25 min	Serving: 12	Beverage pairing: Herbal Tea

Ingredients:

- 1 cup almond flour
- 1/4 cup melted coconut oil
- 1/4 cup sugar-free sweetener (erythritol or stevia)
- 1/2 cup unsweetened shredded coconut
- Zest and juice of 2 lemons
- 3 large eggs
- 1/4 cup coconut flour
- Stevia to taste

Preparation:

1. Preheat the oven to 350°F (175°C) and line a square pan with parchment paper.
2. In a bowl, mix almond flour, melted coconut oil, and sugar-free sweetener to form the crust.
3. Press the crust mixture into the bottom of the lined pan.
4. In another bowl, combine shredded coconut, lemon zest, lemon juice, eggs, coconut flour, and stevia for the lemon coconut layer.
5. Pour the lemon coconut mixture over the crust.
6. Bake for 20-25 minutes or until the edges are golden brown.
7. Allow the bars to cool in the pan for 10 minutes before transferring them to a wire rack.

Nutrient Facts (per lemon bar - makes approximately 12):

- Calories: 100
- Carbohydrates: 5g
- Fat: 8g
- Protein: 3g

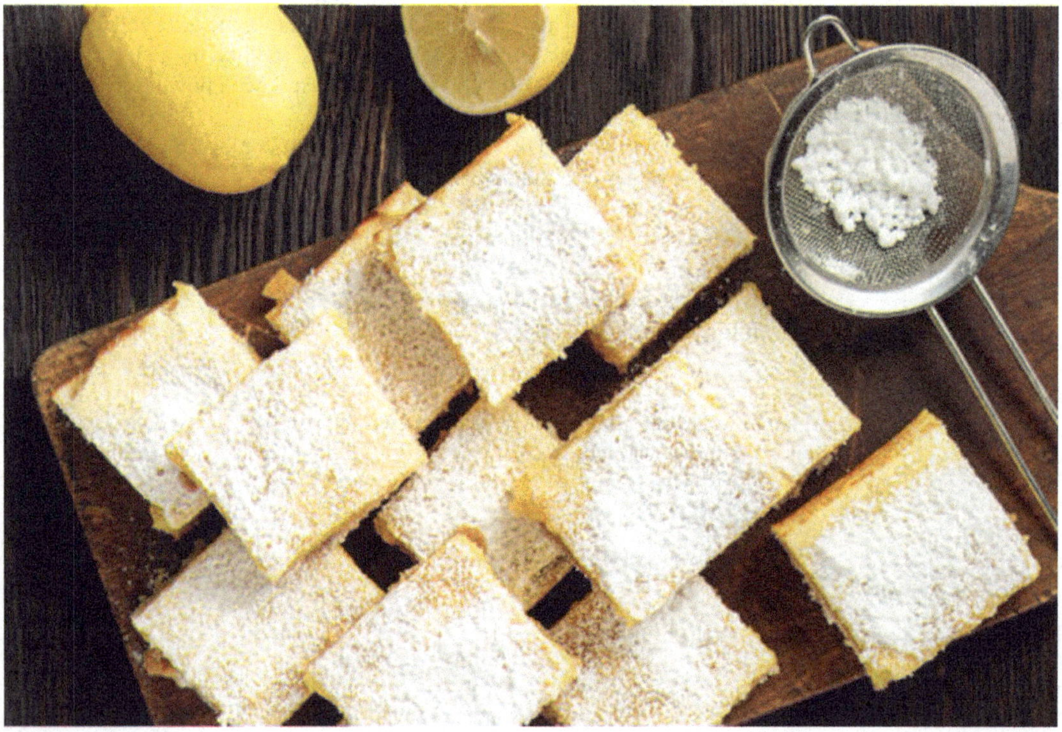

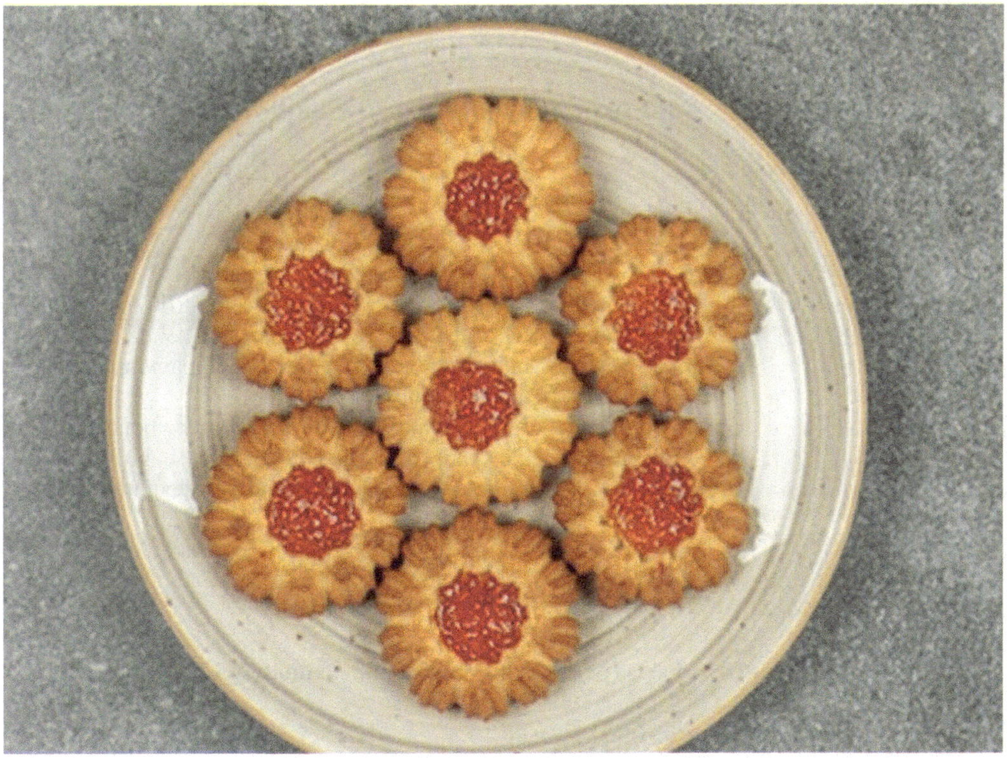

83. Almond Flour Raspberry Thumbprint Cookies

Prep.Time:	Cook Time:	Serving:	Beverage pairing:
15 min	12 min	12	Black Tea

Ingredients:

- 1 cup almond flour
- 1/4 cup melted coconut oil
- 1/4 cup sugar-free sweetener (erythritol or stevia)
- 1 teaspoon vanilla extract
- 1/4 teaspoon almond extract
- A pinch of salt
- Sugar-free raspberry jam

Preparation:

1. Preheat the oven to 350°F (175°C) and line a baking sheet with parchment paper.
2. In a bowl, mix almond flour, melted coconut oil, sugar-free sweetener, vanilla extract, almond extract, and a pinch of salt until well combined.
3. Scoop spoonfuls of the dough onto the prepared baking sheet.
4. Make an indentation in the center of each cookie with your thumb.
5. Fill each indentation with sugar-free raspberry jam.
6. Bake for 10-12 minutes or until the edges are golden brown.
7. Allow the cookies to cool on the baking sheet for 5 minutes before transferring them to a wire rack.

Nutrient Facts (per cookie - makes approximately 12):

- Calories: 80
- Carbohydrates: 3g
- Fat: 7g
- Protein: 2g

84. Coconut Flour Carrot Cake Muffins

Prep.Time:	Cook Time:	Serving:	Beverage pairing:
15 min	25 min	12	Green Tea

Ingredients:

- 1 cup coconut flour
- 1/2 cup shredded carrots
- 1/4 cup melted coconut oil
- 1/4 cup sugar-free sweetener (erythritol or stevia)
- 3 large eggs
- 1 teaspoon vanilla extract
- 1/2 teaspoon ground cinnamon
- 1/4 teaspoon baking soda
- A pinch of salt
- Chopped walnuts for topping (optional)

Preparation:

1. Preheat the oven to 350°F (175°C) and line a muffin tin with paper liners.
2. In a bowl, mix coconut flour, shredded carrots, melted coconut oil, sugar-free sweetener, eggs, vanilla extract, ground cinnamon, baking soda, and a pinch of salt until well combined.
3. Spoon the batter into the muffin cups, filling each about 2/3 full.
4. Optional: Sprinkle chopped walnuts on top of each muffin.
5. Bake for 20-25 minutes or until a toothpick inserted into the center comes out clean.
6. Allow the muffins to cool in the tin for 5 minutes before transferring them to a wire rack to cool completely.

Nutrient Facts (per muffin - makes approximately 12):

- Calories: 100
- Carbohydrates: 6g
- Fat: 7g
- Protein: 3g

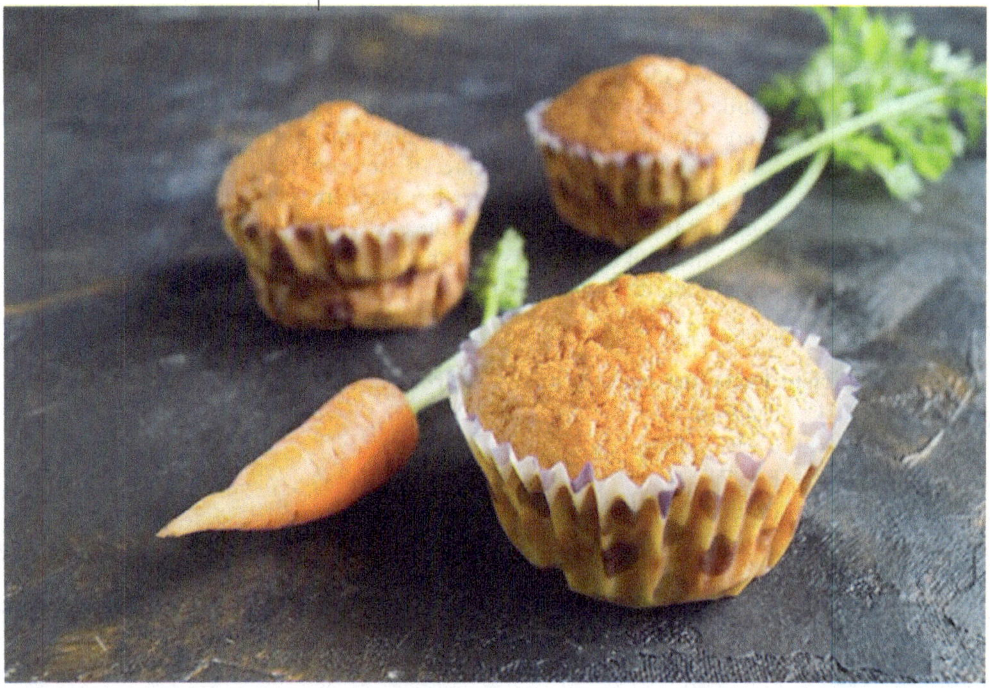

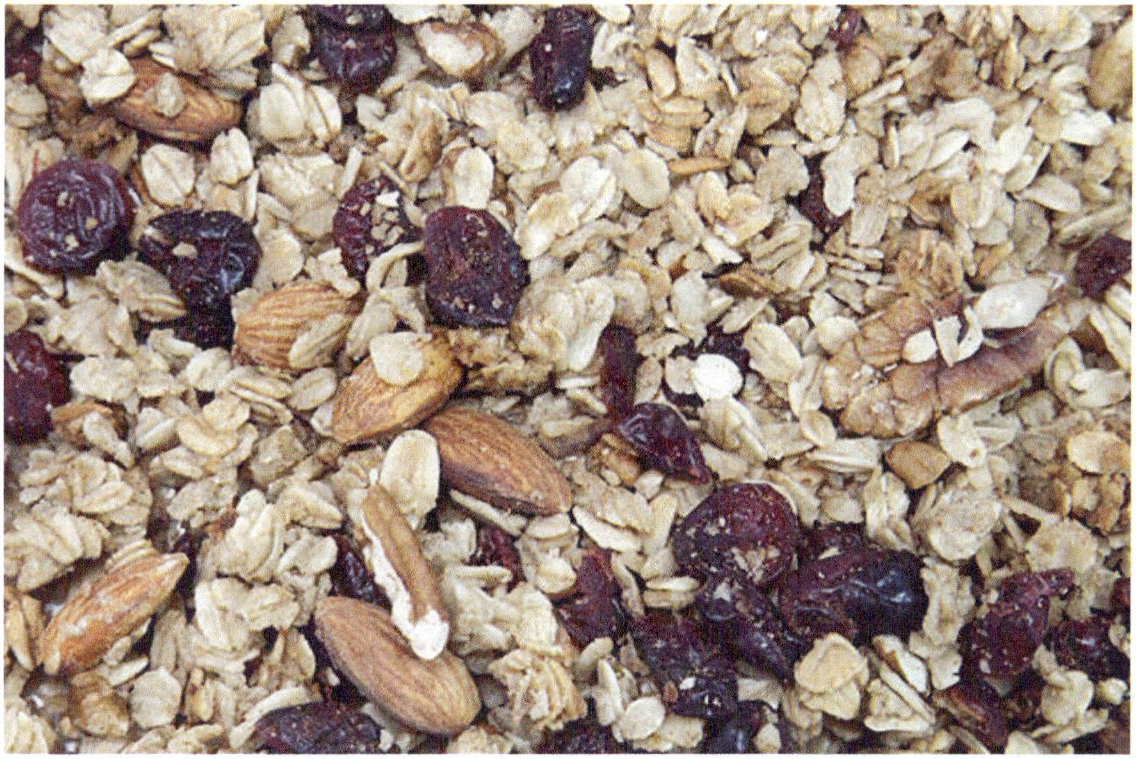

85. Cherry Almond Granola

Prep.Time:	**Cook Time:**	**Serving:**	**Beverage pairing:**
10 min	25 min	8	Herbal Tea

Ingredients:

- 2 cups rolled oats
- 1/2 cup chopped almonds
- 1/4 cup melted coconut oil
- 1/4 cup sugar-free sweetener (erythritol or stevia)
- 1 teaspoon almond extract
- A pinch of salt
- 1/2 cup dried cherries (unsweetened)

Preparation:

1. Preheat the oven to 300°F (150°C) and line a baking sheet with parchment paper.
2. In a bowl, mix rolled oats, chopped almonds, melted coconut oil, sugar-free sweetener, almond extract, and a pinch of salt until well combined.
3. Spread the mixture evenly on the prepared baking sheet.
4. Bake for 20-25 minutes, stirring halfway through, until golden brown.
5. Allow the granola to cool on the baking sheet.
6. Once cooled, mix in dried cherries and break the granola into clusters.

Nutrient Facts (per 1/2 cup serving - makes approximately 8 servings):

- Calories: 150
- Carbohydrates: 14g
- Fat: 9g
- Protein: 3g

86. Avocado Lime Chia Seed Parfait

Prep.Time:	Cook Time:	Serving:	Beverage pairing:
10 min	0 min	2	Coffee

Ingredients:

- 2 ripe avocados
- Zest and juice of 2 limes
- 1/4 cup unsweetened almond milk
- 1/4 cup sugar-free sweetener (erythritol or stevia)
- Stevia to taste
- 1/4 cup chia seeds
- 1 cup unsweetened almond milk

Preparation:

1. In a blender or food processor, blend ripe avocados, lime zest, lime juice, almond milk, and sugar-free sweetener until smooth.
2. Adjust sweetness with more stevia if needed.
3. In a bowl, whisk together chia seeds and almond milk for the chia seed layer.
4. Refrigerate both mixtures for at least 2 hours or until set.
5. Layer the avocado lime pudding and chia seed mixture in serving glasses.

Nutrient Facts (per parfait - serves approximately 2):

- Calories: 200
- Carbohydrates: 14g
- Fat: 15g
- Protein: 5g

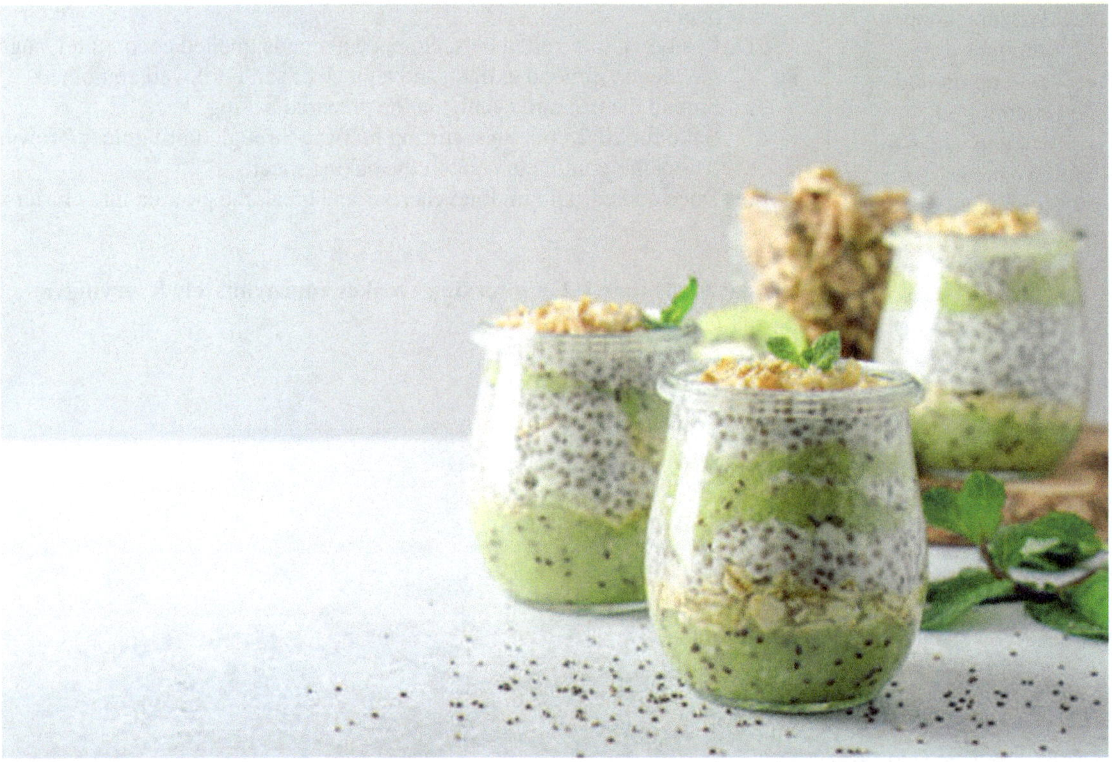

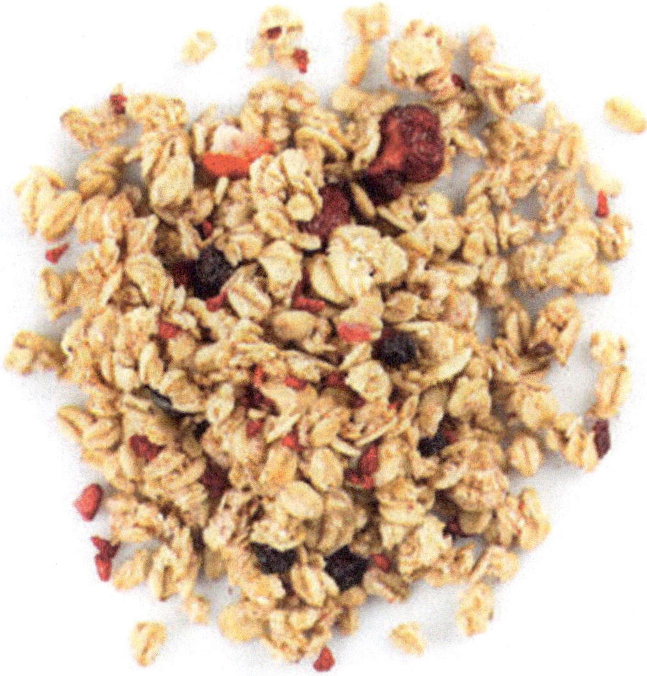

87. Sugar-Free Berry Cobbler

Prep.Time:	Cook Time:	Serving:	Beverage pairing:
15 min	30 min	6	Herbal Tea

Ingredients:

- 2 cups mixed berries (strawberries, blueberries, raspberries)
- 1/4 cup sugar-free sweetener (erythritol or stevia)
- 1 tablespoon lemon juice
- 1 tablespoon arrowroot powder
- 1 cup almond flour
- 1/4 cup melted coconut oil
- 1/4 cup sugar-free sweetener
- 1 teaspoon vanilla extract
- 1/2 teaspoon baking powder
- A pinch of salt

Preparation:

1. Preheat the oven to 350°F (175°C) and grease a baking dish.
2. In a bowl, mix mixed berries, sugar-free sweetener, lemon juice, and arrowroot powder for the berry filling. Transfer the mixture to the prepared baking dish.
3. In another bowl, combine almond flour, melted coconut oil, sugar-free sweetener, vanilla extract, baking powder, and a pinch of salt for the cobbler topping.
4. Drop spoonfuls of the cobbler topping over the berry filling.
5. Bake for 25-30 minutes or until the topping is golden brown.
6. Allow the cobbler to cool for 10 minutes before serving.

Nutrient Facts (per serving - serves approximately 6):

- Calories: 150
- Carbohydrates: 10g
- Fat: 12g
- Protein: 3g

88. Cinnamon Roasted Walnut Clusters

Prep.Time:	Cook Time:	Serving:	Beverage pairing:
5 min	25 min	8	Herbal Tea

Ingredients:

- 2 cups raw walnuts
- 1/4 cup melted coconut oil
- 1/4 cup sugar-free sweetener (erythritol or stevia)
- 1 teaspoon ground cinnamon
- A pinch of salt

Preparation:

1. Preheat the oven to 300°F (150°C) and line a baking sheet with parchment paper.
2. In a bowl, mix raw walnuts, melted coconut oil, sugar-free sweetener, ground cinnamon, and a pinch of salt until well combined.
3. Spread the mixture evenly on the prepared baking sheet.
4. Bake for 20-25 minutes, stirring halfway through, until the walnuts are toasted.
5. Allow the walnut clusters to cool on the baking sheet before serving.

Nutrient Facts (per 1/4 cup serving - makes approximately 8 servings):

- Calories: 180
- Carbohydrates: 3g
- Fat: 18g
- Protein: 4g

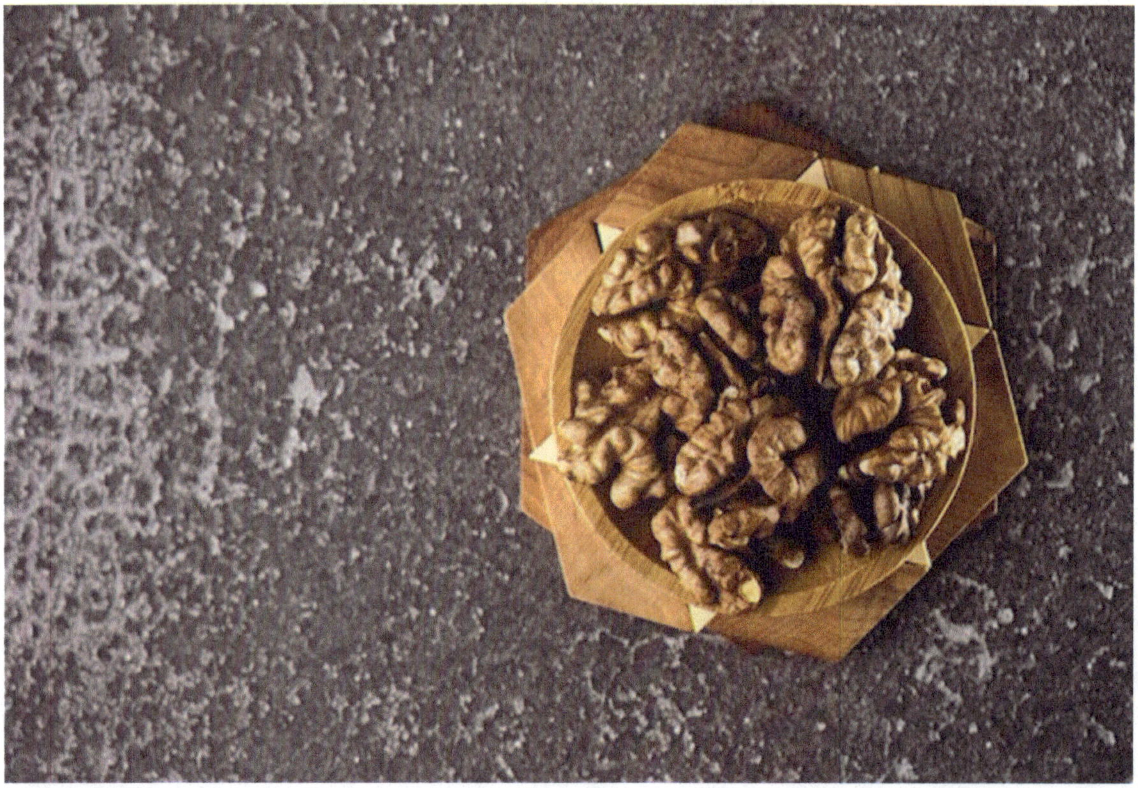

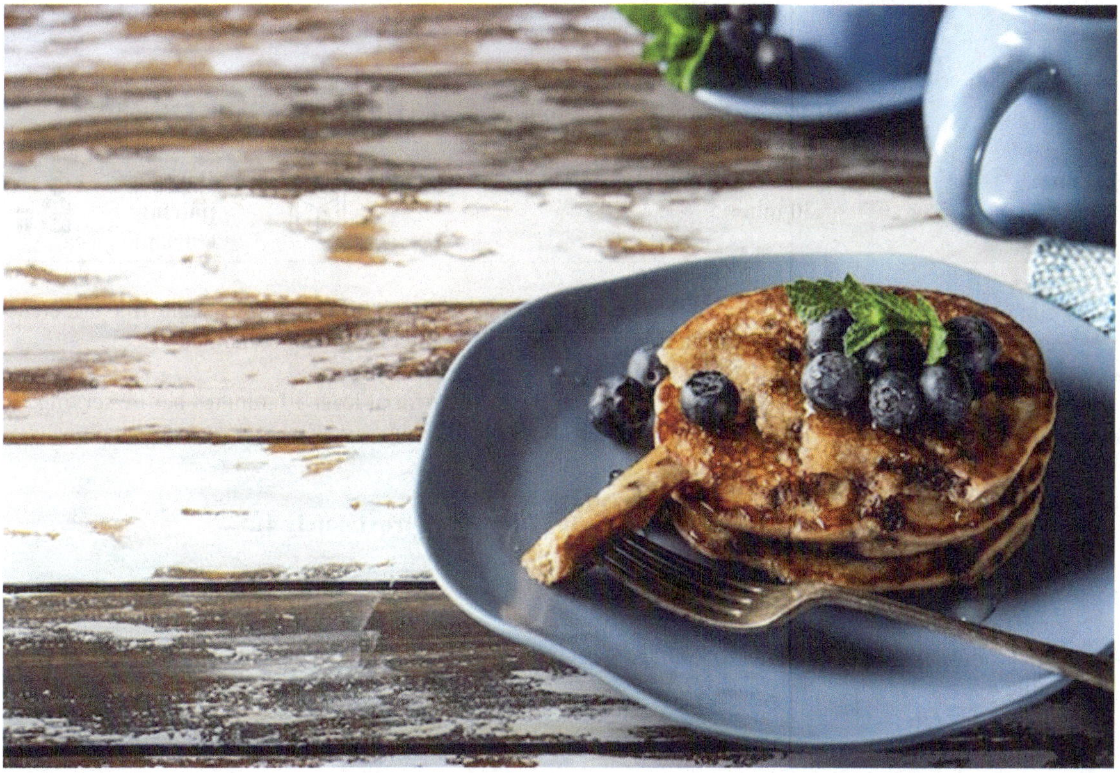

89. Blueberry Almond Coconut Flour Pancakes

Prep.Time: 15 min | **Cook Time:** 10 min | **Serving:** 2 | **Beverage pairing:** Herbal Tea

Ingredients:

- 1/2 cup coconut flour
- 1/2 cup almond flour
- 1 teaspoon baking powder
- 1/4 teaspoon salt
- 3 large eggs
- 1 cup almond milk
- 1 teaspoon vanilla extract
- 1/2 cup fresh blueberries
- Coconut oil for cooking

Preparation:

1. In a bowl, whisk together coconut flour, almond flour, baking powder, and salt.
2. In another bowl, beat the eggs and then add almond milk and vanilla extract. Mix well.
3. Combine the wet and dry ingredients and mix until a smooth batter forms.
4. Gently fold in fresh blueberries.
5. Heat a skillet or griddle over medium heat and add coconut oil.
6. Spoon the batter onto the skillet to form pancakes.
7. Cook until bubbles form on the surface, then flip and cook the other side.
8. Serve with additional blueberries on top.

Nutrient Facts (per serving - makes approximately 4 pancakes):

- Calories: 200
- Carbohydrates: 14g
- Fat: 14g
- Protein: 8g

90. Pumpkin Spice Greek Yogurt Dip with Apple Slices

Prep.Time: 5 min

Cook Time: 30 min

Serving: 4

Beverage pairing: Cinnamon Tea

Ingredients:

- 1 cup plain Greek yogurt
- 1/2 cup canned pumpkin puree
- 2 tablespoons sugar-free sweetener (erythritol or stevia)
- 1 teaspoon pumpkin spice
- 1/2 teaspoon vanilla extract
- Apple slices for dipping

Preparation:

1. In a bowl, mix plain Greek yogurt, pumpkin puree, sugar-free sweetener, pumpkin spice, and vanilla extract until well combined.
2. Adjust sweetness with more stevia if needed.
3. Chill the dip in the refrigerator for at least 30 minutes before serving.
4. Serve with apple slices for dipping.

Nutrient Facts (per serving - serves approximately 4):

- Calories: 70
- Carbohydrates: 8g
- Fat: 2g
- Protein: 5g

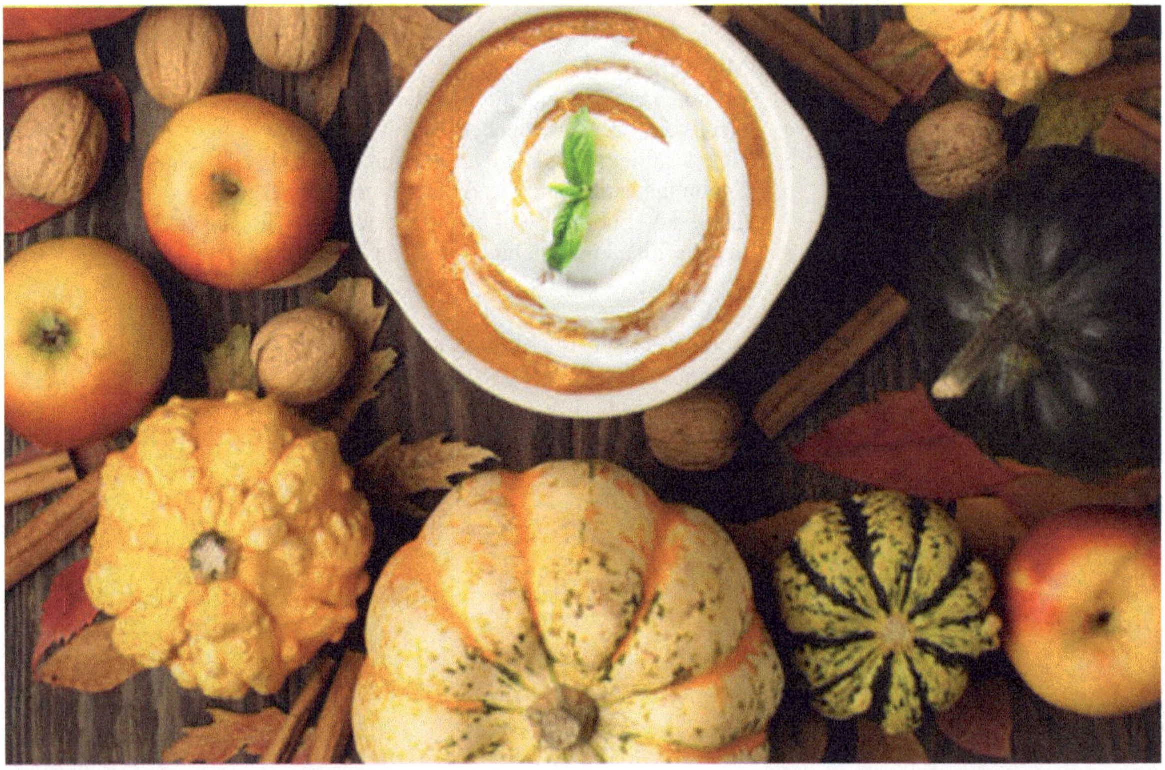

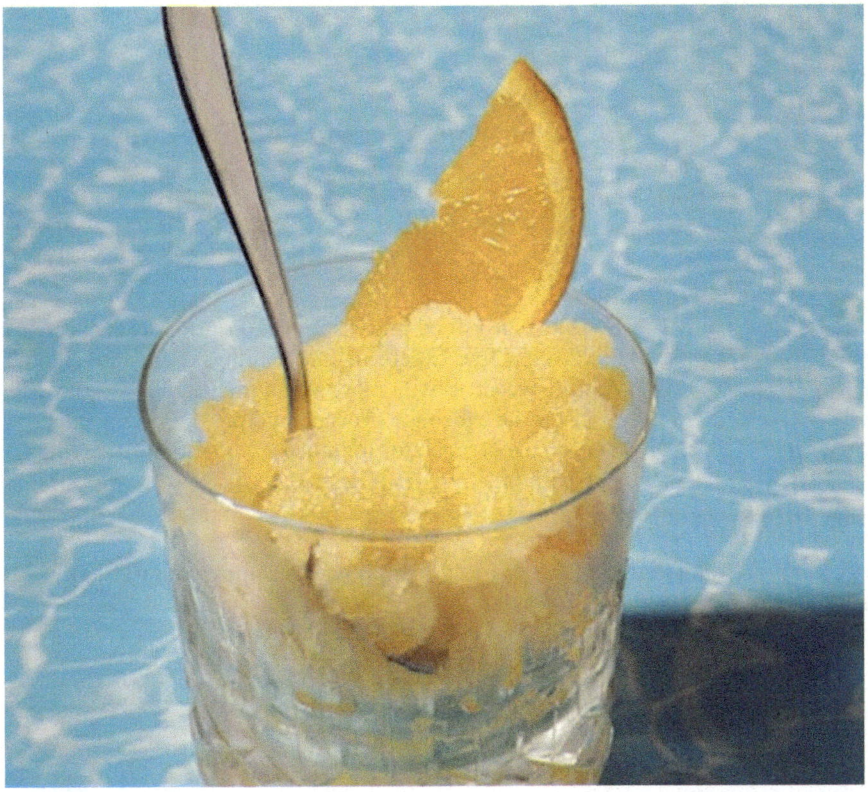

91. No-Sugar Added Mango Lime Sorbet

Prep.Time:	Cook Time:	Serving:	Beverage pairing:
5 min	0 min	2	Lemonade

Ingredients:

- 2 cups frozen mango chunks
- 1/4 cup lime juice
- Zest of 1 lime
- 1/4 cup unsweetened coconut milk
- Stevia to taste

Preparation:

1. In a blender or food processor, blend frozen mango chunks, lime juice, lime zest, and unsweetened coconut milk until smooth.
2. Adjust sweetness with more stevia if needed.
3. Transfer the mixture to a shallow dish and freeze for at least 4 hours, stirring every hour.
4. Once fully frozen, scoop out the sorbet and serve.

Nutrient Facts (per serving - serves approximately 2):

- Calories: 100
- Carbohydrates: 24g
- Fat: 1g
- Protein: 1g

92. Chocolate Avocado Pudding Cups

Prep.Time:	Cook Time:	Serving:	Beverage pairing:
10 min	0 min	2	Black Tea

Ingredients:

- 2 ripe avocados
- 1/4 cup unsweetened cocoa powder
- 1/4 cup almond milk
- 1/4 cup sugar-free sweetener (erythritol or stevia)
- 1 teaspoon vanilla extract
- Stevia to taste
- Fresh berries for topping (optional)

Preparation:

1. In a blender or food processor, blend ripe avocados, cocoa powder, almond milk, sugar-free sweetener, and vanilla extract until smooth.
2. Adjust sweetness with more stevia if needed.
3. Transfer the chocolate avocado pudding to serving cups.
4. Chill in the refrigerator for at least 1 hour before serving.
5. Top with fresh berries if desired.

Nutrient Facts (per pudding cup - serves approximately 2):

- Calories: 200
- Carbohydrates: 15g
- Fat: 16g
- Protein: 4g

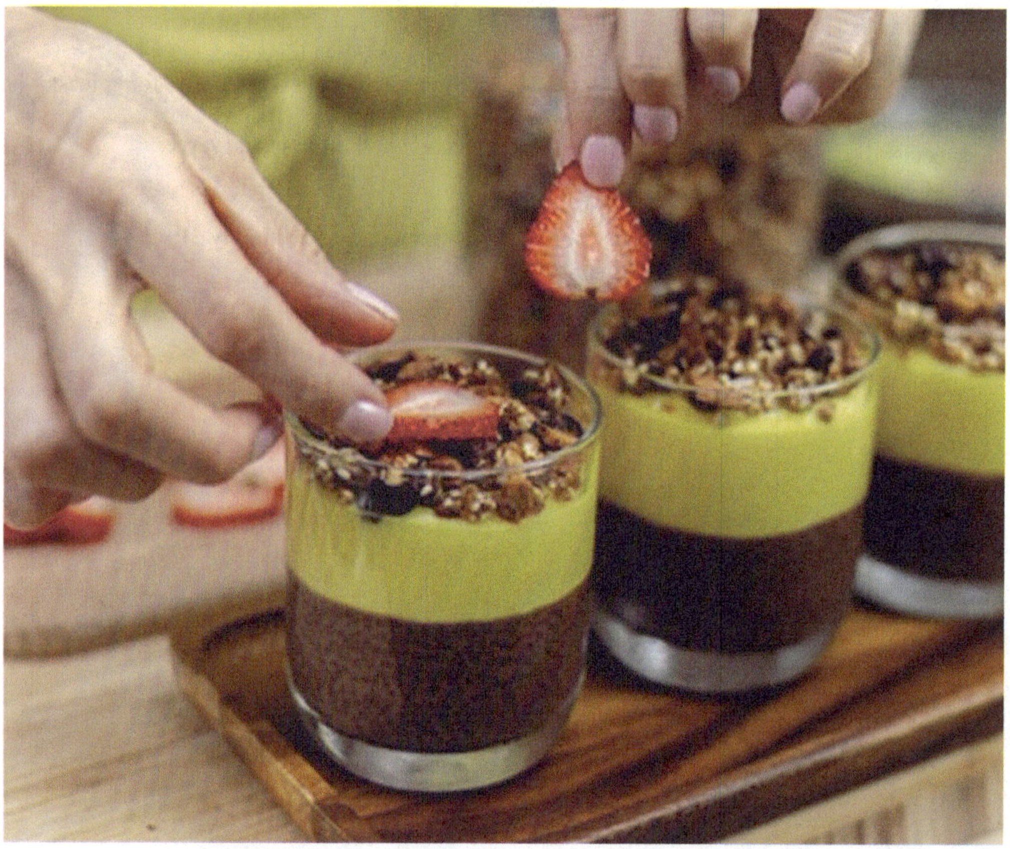

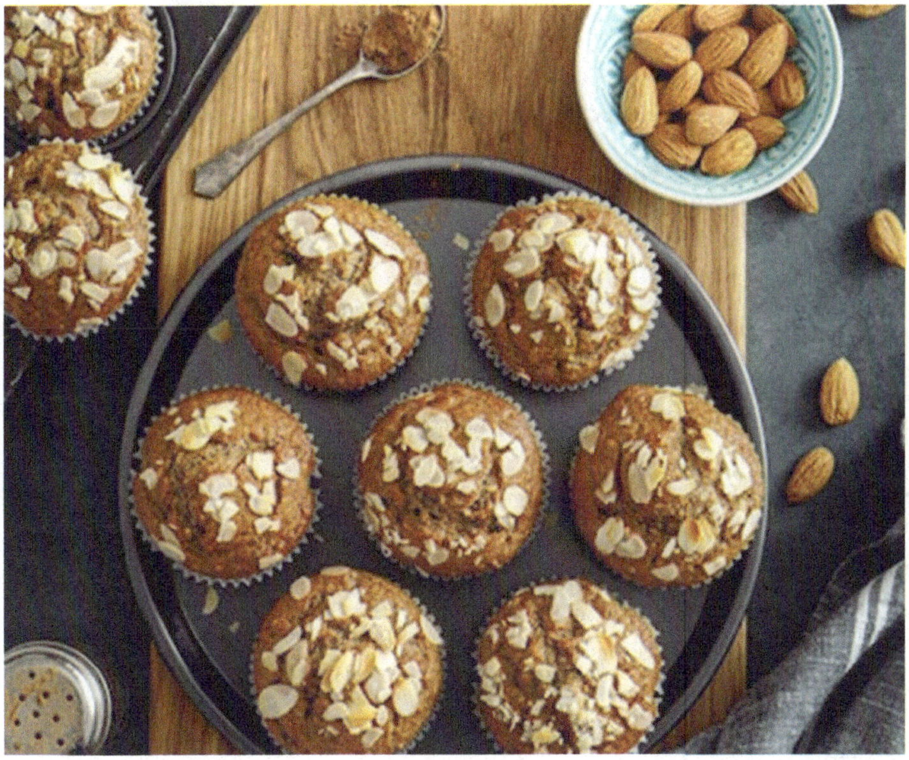

93. Almond Flour Banana Walnut Muffins

Prep.Time: 15 min

Cook Time: 25 min

Serving: 12

Beverage pairing: Green Tea

Ingredients:

- 2 cups almond flour
- 1/4 cup melted coconut oil
- 1/4 cup sugar-free sweetener (erythritol or stevia)
- 3 ripe bananas, mashed
- 3 large eggs
- 1 teaspoon vanilla extract
- 1/2 teaspoon baking soda
- A pinch of salt
- 1/2 cup chopped walnuts

Preparation:

1. Preheat the oven to 350°F (175°C) and line a muffin tin with paper liners.
2. In a bowl, mix almond flour, melted coconut oil, sugar-free sweetener, mashed bananas, eggs, vanilla extract, baking soda, and a pinch of salt until well combined.
3. Fold in chopped walnuts.
4. Spoon the batter into the muffin cups, filling each about 2/3 full.
5. Bake for 20-25 minutes or until a toothpick inserted into the center comes out clean.
6. Allow the muffins to cool in the tin for 5 minutes before transferring them to a wire rack to cool completely.

Nutrient Facts (per muffin - makes approximately 12):

- Calories: 150
- Carbohydrates: 10g
- Fat: 11g
- Protein: 5g

94. Berry Coconut Chia Seed Smoothie Bowl

Prep.Time: 5 min | **Cook Time:** 0 min | **Serving:** 1 | **Beverage pairing:** Herbal Tea

Ingredients:

- 1 cup mixed berries (strawberries, blueberries, raspberries)
- 1/2 frozen banana
- 1/4 cup unsweetened coconut milk
- 2 tablespoons chia seeds
- Stevia to taste
- Fresh berries
- Unsweetened shredded coconut
- Chopped nuts

Preparation:

1. In a blender, blend mixed berries, frozen banana, unsweetened coconut milk, and chia seeds until smooth.
2. Adjust sweetness with more stevia if needed.
3. Pour the smoothie into a bowl.
4. Top with fresh berries, shredded coconut, and chopped nuts.

Nutrient Facts (per smoothie bowl):

- Calories: 250
- Carbohydrates: 30g
- Fat: 10g
- Protein: 5g

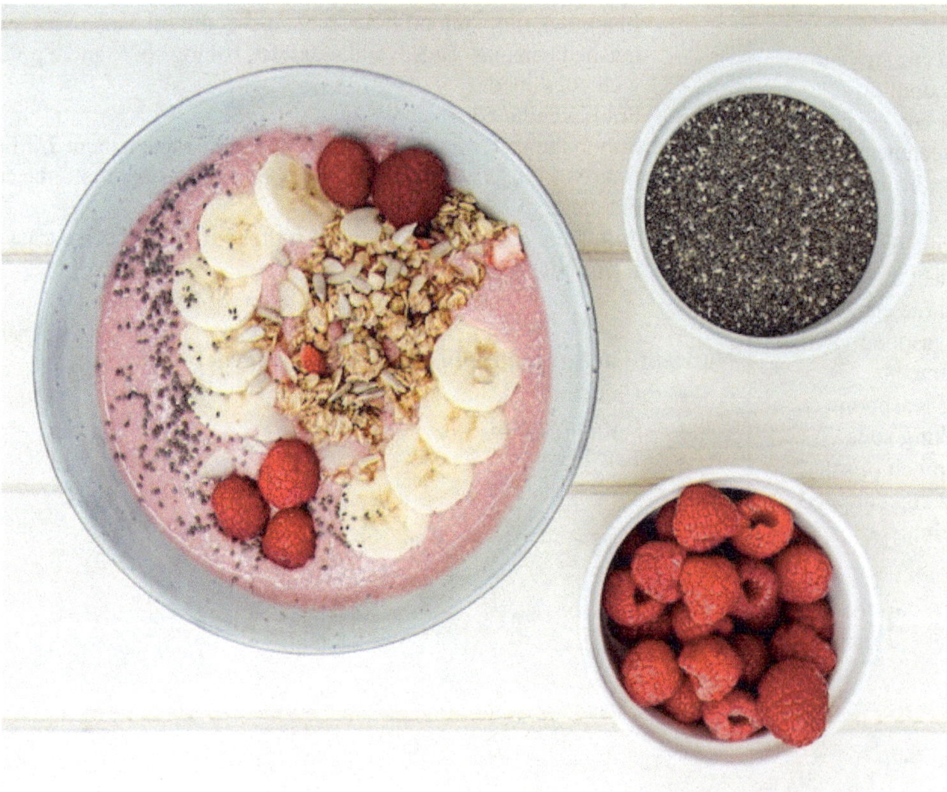

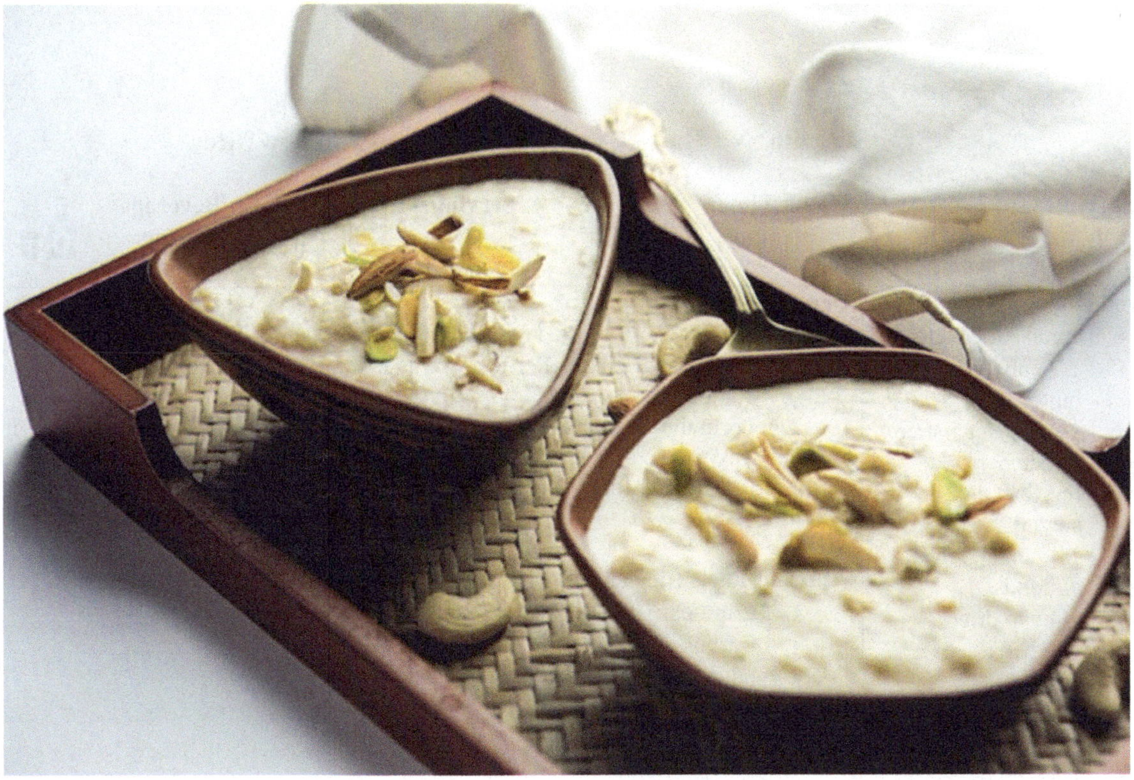

95. Vanilla Cashew Milk Rice Pudding

Prep.Time: 10 min

Cook Time: 15 min

Serving: 4

Beverage pairing: Herbal Tea

Ingredients:

- 1 cup cooked white rice
- 2 cups unsweetened cashew milk
- 1/4 cup sugar-free sweetener (erythritol or stevia)
- 1 teaspoon vanilla extract
- A pinch of salt
- Ground cinnamon for topping

Preparation:

1. In a saucepan, combine cooked white rice, unsweetened cashew milk, sugar-free sweetener, vanilla extract, and a pinch of salt.
2. Cook over medium heat, stirring frequently, until the mixture thickens.
3. Remove from heat and let it cool slightly.
4. Transfer the rice pudding to serving bowls and sprinkle ground cinnamon on top.

Nutrient Facts (per serving - serves approximately 4):

- Calories: 120
- Carbohydrates: 20g
- Fat: 3g
- Protein: 2g

96. No-Bake Cranberry Almond Energy Bites

Prep.Time: 15 min	**Cook Time:** 30 min	**Serving:** 12	**Beverage pairing:** Herbal Tea

Ingredients:

- 1 cup rolled oats
- 1/2 cup almond butter
- 1/4 cup sugar-free sweetener (erythritol or stevia)
- 1/4 cup chopped almonds
- 1/4 cup dried cranberries (unsweetened)
- 1 teaspoon vanilla extract
- A pinch of salt

Preparation:

1. In a bowl, mix rolled oats, almond butter, sugar-free sweetener, chopped almonds, dried cranberries, vanilla extract, and a pinch of salt until well combined.
2. Form the mixture into bite-sized balls and place them on a parchment-lined tray.
3. Refrigerate for at least 30 minutes before serving.

Nutrient Facts (per energy bite - makes approximately 12):

- Calories: 100
- Carbohydrates: 10g
- Fat: 6g
- Protein: 3g

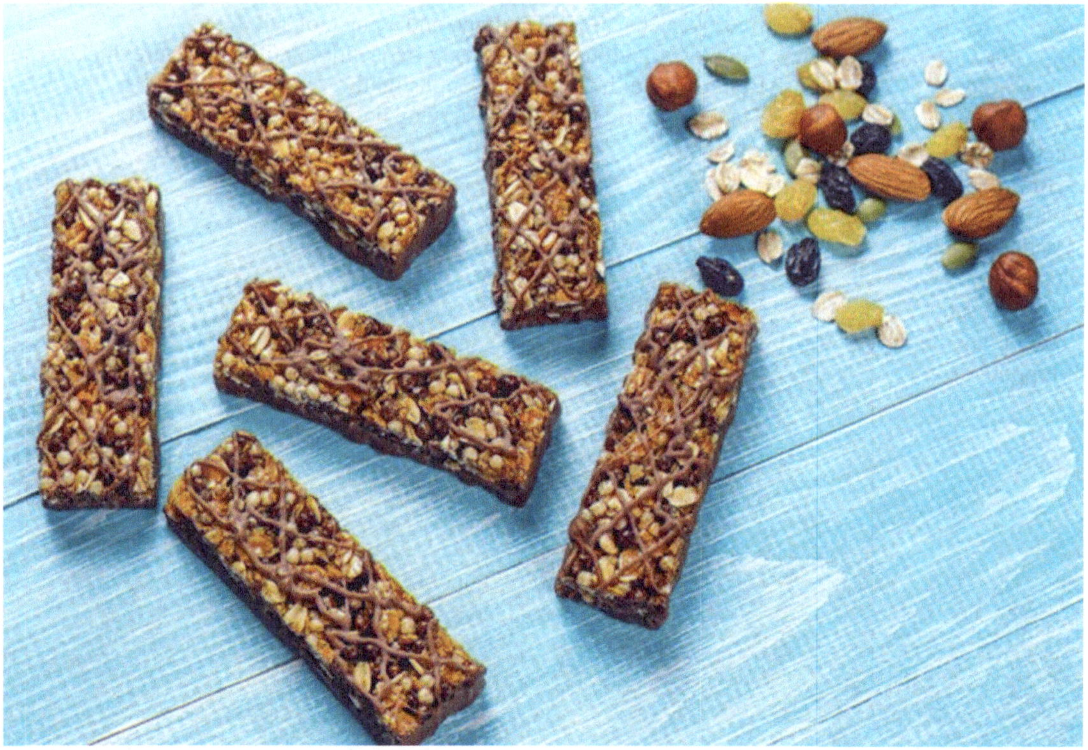

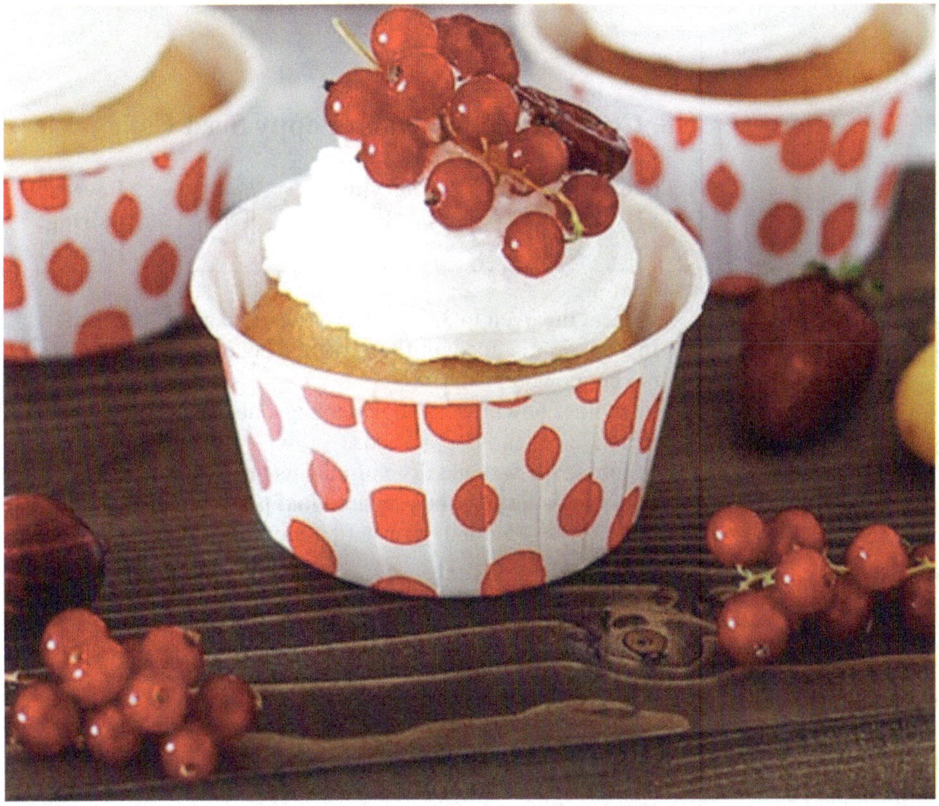

97. Sugar-Free Lemon Raspberry Cheesecake Cups

Prep.Time:	**Cook Time:**	**Serving:**	**Beverage pairing:**
20 min	20 min	12	Black Tea

Ingredients:

- 1 cup almond flour
- 1/4 cup melted coconut oil
- 1/4 cup sugar-free sweetener (erythritol or stevia)
- 1 cup cream cheese, softened
- 1/4 cup sugar-free sweetener
- 1 teaspoon vanilla extract
- Zest and juice of 1 lemon
- Stevia to taste
- 1/2 cup fresh raspberries

Preparation:

1. Preheat the oven to 350°F (175°C) and line a muffin tin with paper liners.
2. In a bowl, mix almond flour, melted coconut oil, and sugar-free sweetener to form the crust.
3. Press the crust mixture into the bottom of each muffin cup.
4. In another bowl, beat together cream cheese, sugar-free sweetener, vanilla extract, lemon zest, lemon juice, and stevia until smooth.
5. Spoon the cheesecake filling over the crust in each muffin cup.
6. In a small saucepan, heat fresh raspberries with stevia until they release their juices.
7. Mash the raspberries and spoon the topping over the cheesecake filling.
8. Bake for 15-20 minutes or until set.
9. Allow the cheesecake cups to cool in the tin for 10 minutes before transferring them to a wire rack.

Nutrient Facts (per cheesecake cup - makes approximately 12):

- Calories: 120
- Carbohydrates: 5g
- Fat: 10g
- Protein: 3g

98. Coconut Flour Lemon Poppy Seed Cake

Prep.Time:	Cook Time:	Serving:	Beverage pairing:
15 min	45 min	10	Herbal Tea

Ingredients:

- 1 cup coconut flour
- 1/2 cup melted coconut oil
- 1/4 cup sugar-free sweetener (erythritol or stevia)
- 1 teaspoon baking powder
- 1/4 teaspoon salt
- 4 large eggs
- 1 cup unsweetened almond milk
- Zest and juice of 1 lemon
- 1 tablespoon poppy seeds
- 1/4 cup coconut cream
- 1 tablespoon lemon juice

Preparation:

1. Preheat the oven to 350°F (175°C) and grease a loaf pan.
2. In a bowl, mix coconut flour, melted coconut oil, sugar-free sweetener, baking powder, and salt.
3. In another bowl, whisk together eggs, unsweetened almond milk, lemon zest, lemon juice, and poppy seeds.
4. Combine the wet and dry ingredients until well combined.
5. Pour the batter into the prepared loaf pan.
6. Bake for 40-45 minutes or until a toothpick inserted into the center comes out clean.
7. In a small saucepan, heat coconut cream, lemon juice, and stevia for the glaze.
8. Drizzle the glaze over the cooled cake.

Nutrient Facts (per slice - serves approximately 10):

- Calories: 150
- Carbohydrates: 8g
- Fat: 11g
- Protein: 4g

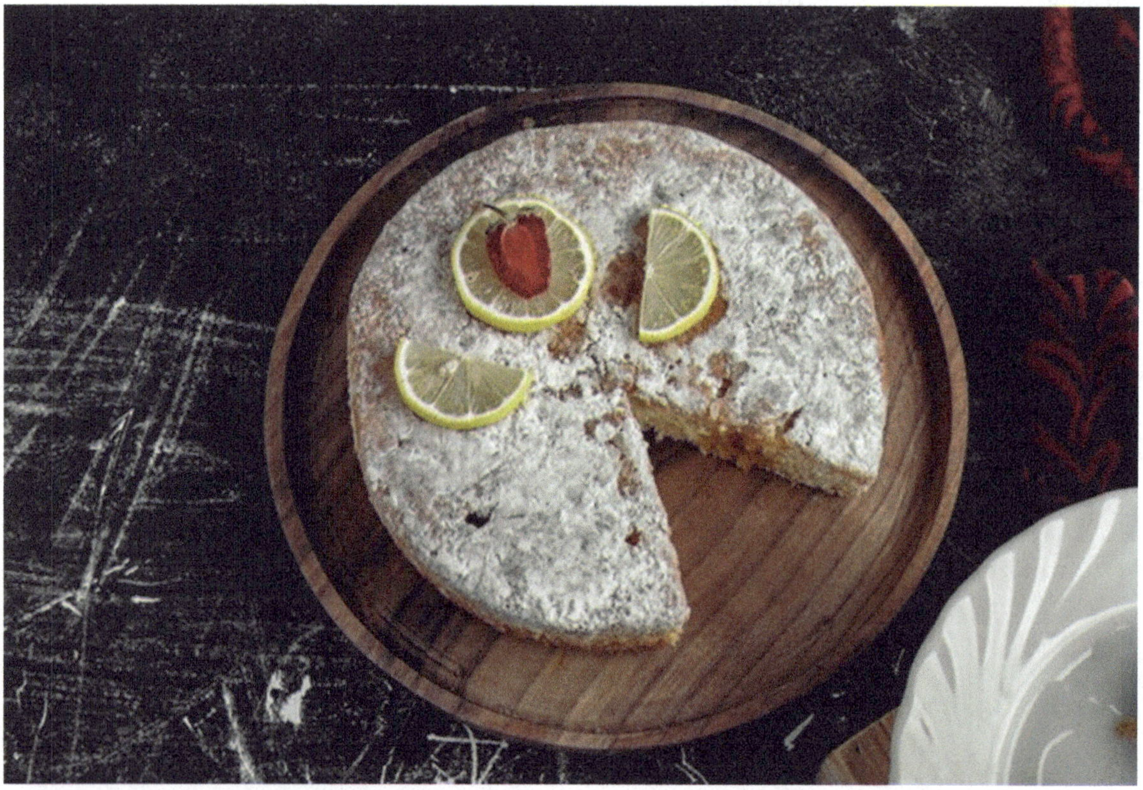

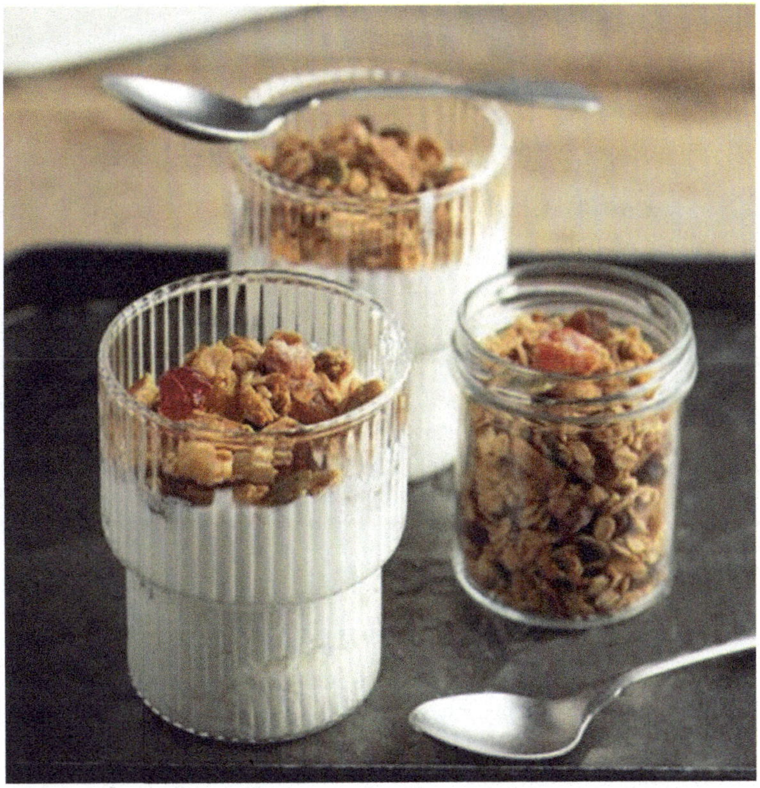

99. Pecan Pie Greek Yogurt Parfait

Prep.Time: 5 min

Cook Time: 0 min

Serving: 2

Beverage pairing: Coffee

Ingredients:

- 1 cup plain Greek yogurt
- 1 tablespoon sugar-free sweetener (erythritol or stevia)
- 1/4 cup chopped **pecans**
- 1/2 teaspoon vanilla extract
- 1 tablespoon sugar-free caramel sauce

Preparation:

1. In a bowl, mix plain Greek yogurt, sugar-free sweetener, chopped **pecans**, and vanilla extract.
2. In serving glasses, layer the Greek yogurt mixture with drizzles of sugar-free caramel sauce.
3. Repeat the layers until the glass is filled.
4. Top with additional chopped **pecans** and a final drizzle of caramel sauce.

Nutrient Facts (per parfait - serves approximately 2):

- Calories: 200
- Carbohydrates: 10g
- Fat: 15g
- Protein: 10g

100. Cocoa-Dusted Hazelnut Clusters

Prep.Time:	Cook Time:	Serving:	Beverage pairing:
5 min	25 min	8	Herbal Tea

Ingredients:

- 2 cups raw hazelnuts
- 1/4 cup melted coconut oil
- 2 tablespoons unsweetened cocoa powder
- 1/4 cup sugar-free sweetener (erythritol or stevia)
- A pinch of salt

Preparation:

1. Preheat the oven to 300°F (150°C) and line a baking sheet with parchment paper.
2. In a bowl, mix raw **hazelnuts**, melted coconut oil, unsweetened cocoa powder, sugar-free sweetener, and a pinch of salt until well combined.
3. Spread the mixture evenly on the prepared baking sheet.
4. Bake for 20-25 minutes, stirring halfway through, until the **hazelnuts** are toasted.
5. Allow the clusters to cool on the baking sheet before serving.

Nutrient Facts (per 1/4 cup serving - makes approximately 8 servings):

- Calories: 180
- Carbohydrates: 4g
- Fat: 17g
- Protein: 4g

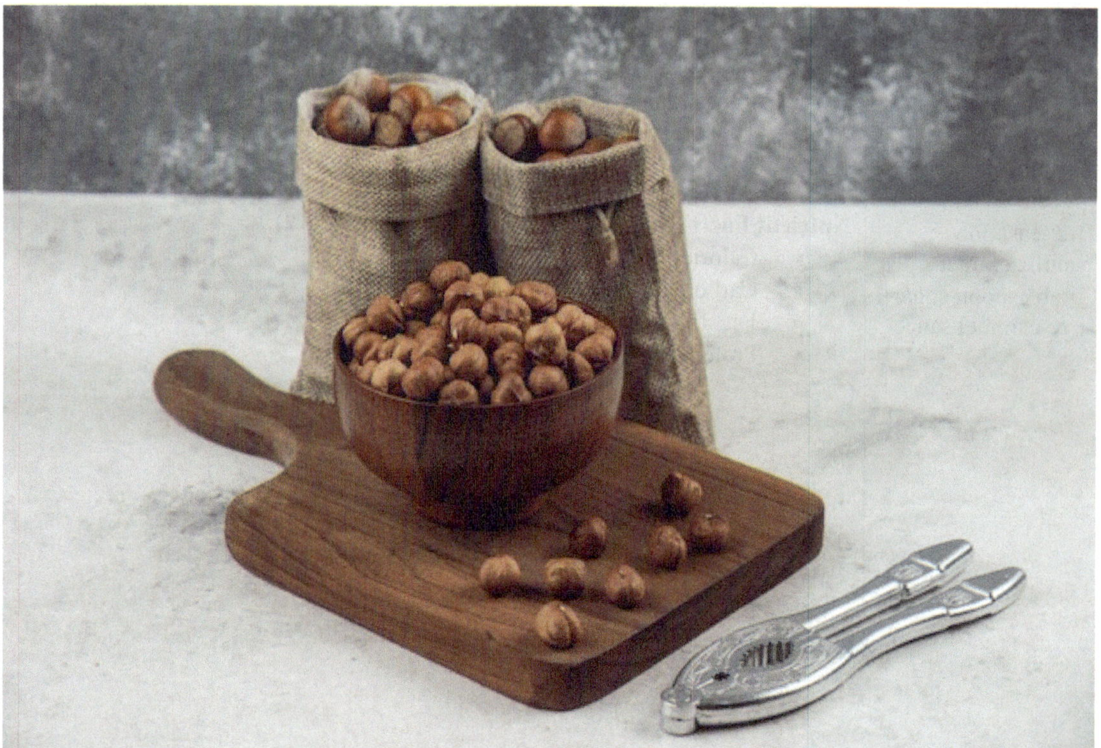

Sharing Your Culinary Journey

Now that you've mastered the art of creating delicious, diabetes-friendly meals, it's time to share your newfound culinary wisdom with others who are on the same path. By leaving your honest review of the "Type 2 Diabetes Cookbook: Beginner's Quick & Easy Recipes for Delicious Diabetes Diets" by Lily Anders on Amazon, you'll guide fellow food enthusiasts to a resource that can transform their dining table and health.

Your insights and experiences are invaluable, offering a beacon to those navigating their diet amidst diabetes. Whether it was a specific recipe that became your go-to, a tip that changed how you approach cooking, or the overall ease and enjoyment you found in these pages, your feedback is a gift that keeps on giving.

Thank you for contributing to a community of knowledge and support. The journey towards healthy eating and diabetes management thrives on shared discoveries and successes. By passing on your review, you're not just recommending a book—you're enriching lives with the joy of cooking and the empowerment of dietary control.

To leave your review, just follow this link:

https://www.amazon.com/review/create-review/?ie=UTF8&channel=glance-detail&asin=1963939328

Together, we're keeping the passion for healthy, joyful eating alive, one review at a time. Your support makes all the difference, not just to us, but to every reader and cook who seeks to balance their love for food with their health needs.

- With heartfelt thanks,

Lily Anders

Conclusion

In conclusion, this book transcends the traditional approach to managing diabetes through diet alone, offering a comprehensive guide that empowers individuals with diabetes to navigate their condition with knowledge and precision. Through 300 carefully crafted recipes, we explore the importance of balancing nutrient intake and the vital role of consistent meal planning. Each recipe is not just a set of instructions but a building block towards a healthier life, tailored to the unique needs of those managing diabetes.

As we close this journey of understanding and adaptation, remember that managing diabetes is not just about adhering to dietary restrictions or grappling with numbers—it is about reclaiming control of your health and life. These recipes are designed not only to meet specific nutritional needs but also to delight the palate, proving that a diabetes-conscious diet can be as delicious as it is nutritious.

Embrace these culinary tools as your allies in the pursuit of wellness. Let each meal enrich your body and spirit, and may the knowledge contained in this book guide you toward a balanced, joyful, and healthy life with diabetes. Here's to finding pleasure in every bite and strength in every challenge. Cheers to your health and happiness on this flavorful journey!

Made in the USA
Coppell, TX
22 August 2026

87800870R00077